Devastated

Devastated

How gender ideology is tearing
Australian families apart

Edited by
Kirralie Smith

Copyright © 2024 by Gender Awareness Australia Ltd
Printed in Australia

For further information, please write to:
Gender Awareness Australia Ltd
GPO Box 1467
Sydney NSW 2001
Or visit:
www.binary.org.au

All rights reserved. No part of this publication may be reproduced, stored in a retrieval system or transmitted in any form by any means, electronic, mechanical, photocopying, recording or otherwise, without the prior written permission of the publishers and copyright holders.

Devastated
ISBN 978-0-646-70319-0

 A catalogue record for this book is available from the National Library of Australia

Contents

Introduction 7

Jennifer's story 13

Tess's story 17

Tara's story 63

Melinda's story 73

Rachel's story 79

Emma and Paul's story 83

Danielle's story 89

Kelly's story 93

Natalie's story 99

How did the media get it so wrong? 127

Dianna Kenny — a practitioner's perspective 135

The international and Australian context 143

Resources for families 153

The future for our children 159

Introduction

Gender identity ideology is destroying families in Australia.

I understand that is a big statement to make. It sounds dramatic and dangerous.

That's because it is.

This book contains the first-hand accounts of some of those families. They represent thousands of families in the same situation right now.

I have been the spokeswoman and a director for Binary Australia for the past five years. During this time I have received hundreds, if not thousands of messages, emails, phone calls and personal accounts of the way that gender identity ideology has destroyed the lives of young people and their families.

For many it begins with confusing ideas presented to children as young as 3 years old in childcare, library books, movies and television shows.

Many parents complain about the endless parade of special days and programs in their child or grandchild's school that celebrate or promote aspects of gender ideology focused on sexual orientations and sexual identities. Note the word 'sexual'. It is completely inappropriate, and sometimes dangerous, to present sexual concepts to children. They are children! As a society, we have always understood that mature concepts regarding sexuality need to be presented to children in an age appropriate

INTRODUCTION

way. It has always involved the consent of the parents, who are the first and primary educators of their children. Children are not mature enough to be presented with sexual concepts, ideas or activities.

Special days incorporating complex sexual ideas are known by euphemisms that sound harmless, but hide sinister motives. Wear it Purple day, IDOHOBIT day, Rainbow events, Pride days and Pride month, Queer days and coming out days. Every one of these days encourage children to focus on sexual orientations or sexual identities. It is not appropriate to involve children in celebrations of anything 'sexual.'

Parents simply want their children to be educated, to be healthy and well-adjusted members of society. Parents expect schools to do this without introducing or promoting complex sexual concepts to children.

Yet it appears the education system, health system and legal system are actively working against these goals and desires when it comes to gender identity. And subverting parents in the process.

The health system is meant to build upon the adage "do no harm". Yet they are engaging in experimental practices on children by using off-label drugs and unstudied pathways to deal with gender incongruence.

Hamstrung by constrictive legislation, many practitioners are wary of treating the underlying issues that present as gender incongruence because they do not want to be victims of laws that accuse them of transphobia, which can result in a loss of licence to practice.

Dr Jillian Spencer, a senior psychiatrist at the Queensland Children's Hospital found out the hard way that it is not acceptable to even question the use of experimental, off-label use of medications such as puberty blockers. As a result, Dr Spencer has been accused of transphobia and stood down from her role following a complaint made against her.

Other practitioners simply refer their patients on to gender clinics and refuse to address the autism, trauma, depression, abuse or social contagion that has triggered the gender questioning in the first place. They admit that these are the real issues that need to be addressed but lawmakers have made it almost impossible to do so without facing severe penalties.

Western culture is being overrun with 'progressive' ideologies that do not tolerate debate, analysis or opposition.

Activists promoting gender ideology in government, education and health are often loud and very threatening. They claim their ideological views are 'tolerant and inclusive' while actively penalising or threatening those who challenge their views.

Cancel culture is real. It is powerful and effective. As you read the stories in this book, you will understand the dilemma many parents face as a result of the intimidation, legal and social repercussions of opposing this agenda when it comes to their own children.

Parents and teenagers navigating the troubled waters of puberty are facing greater obstacles to healthy development than ever before.

Puberty is a right of passage for every human being. It is the necessary process every person must endure to reach full maturity. A child cannot become an adult without the physical, emotional, mental and social development forged through puberty.

Our identity as adults relies on the formation that happens during puberty.

It is a difficult and sometimes painful period in our lives. It is a time we need the support, guidance and acceptance of trusted and mature adults in our lives. Yet in recent years there has been an explosion in the numbers of young people rejecting this necessary part of their development. Activist adults have not only enabled children to indulge their confusion but they have successfully prohibited responsible adults from supporting confused and hurting children.

Thousands of young autistic or traumatised youth are being offered ways to suppress their development, instead of being supported through it.

There has been an alarming rise in the number of young people identifying as something they are not and never can be! No one can change their sex. A boy cannot become a girl. A girl cannot become a boy.

Social media has created an environment where children explore these complex issues without the nurture and supervision of caring and responsible adults to guide them. Some children are so desperate for acceptance, or to numb their pain that they resort to extreme measures to access what they feel would be a quick fix.

Children and teens are being groomed online to accuse their parents of not being understanding or supportive of their desire to 'transition' to escape their authority and negate the need for consent.

You may be tempted to think that this just happens in broken families or where children are not disciplined. It is simply not true. As you read these accounts you will see this is happening in families just like yours. Families with loving parents and siblings, families of faith and families of no faith, families in the suburbs, families just trying to navigate life the best they can.

Unfortunately we are living in the perfect storm, created by activists over decades, that has seen the legal system, health system and education system converge to undermine parental rights and consent while equipping vulnerable young people with the tools they need to permanently and catastrophically damage their bodies and minds in horrific ways.

Already transgender regret is a growing phenomenon. As children captured by the ideology become adults they realise how deficient they are due to medicalised interventions that have stunted their growth and left them scarred and life-long medical dependents.

It is criminal and sad beyond words.

The growing number of devastated and abandoned young adults must cause us to sit up and take note. There will only be more as the years pass and more children reach adulthood.

Lying to children or to anyone in fact, is not kind. It is cruel to deceive already confused people into believing they can achieve the impossible. Pronouns and name changes will not change a person's sex. Costumes, make-up and hairstyles are simply appropriations of stereotypes. Becoming a lifelong medical patient, reliant on drugs and very risky surgical procedures will not turn a male into a female or a female into a male.

It is devastating to families and children that activists have succeeded in convincing legislators that these lies will result in freedom. They never will. Only the truth will set them free.

As for the phenomenon known as gender fluid or non-binary, it is important to note that no third gamete has ever been discovered. There are only two sexes – male and female. Male and female denote reproductive systems and gametes. There are only two – males are geared around the production of small gametes known as sperm, and females are geared around the production of large gametes, known as eggs. There is no third gamete or reproductive system.

Gender fluid or non-binary is simply a personality preference. There is no problem with being gender non-conforming. So what if a girl likes stereotypical masculine appearances or pursuits? So what if she likes trucks, mechanical engineering or sport? So what if a male embraces feminine stereotypes?

Didn't we spend decades breaking down gender stereotypes so tomboys and feminine males could thrive without judgement or discrimination?

Why are there now some people who insist on medicalising and making those stereotypes permanent? Why shouldn't we continue to encourage young people to express themselves and accept themselves as they are without conforming to such rigid stereotypes?

Very few people have an issue with costumes or make up or even names. It becomes a problem however when activists attempt to convert these confused young people into life-long medical patients propping up a powerful pharmaceutical industry. It becomes a problem when we are all compelled to lie and condone the lie for the sake of someone else's feelings.

We also have to ask why are there some who insist genitals don't determine your gender but then go to great lengths to appear to have the genitals of the opposite sex? Thanks to social media it is not difficult to find horrifying testimonies from those who have surgically removed or refashioned perfectly healthy body parts to now be living a nightmare. Infections, non-functioning genitals, and other complications must serve as serious warning to anyone considering these drastic measures for the sake of appropriating the appearance of the opposite sex.

Gender identity ideology is impacting real lives, real families and way too many children and teenagers in this country. My hope is that as you read this book and share it among your networks, Australian families will become more informed and activated. We must do all we can to protect a generation from irreversible and catastrophic harm.

The only way we can succeed is to raise awareness, be informed and educated. We must lobby those in power, and support those who are caught up in this mess.

My hope is that the stories in this book will inform you, move you and equip you to do just that.

Kirralie Smith

BINARY AUSTRALIA

CHAPTER ONE
Jennifer's story

In the port town of Newcastle in NSW, amidst the hustle and bustle of life, my husband and I found ourselves on an unexpected journey—one that would threaten the health and wellbeing of our daughter and cause untold damage to our family.

On the verge of adulthood at just eighteen, our daughter Sophie declared to us she no longer identified as female and that she suddenly wanted to be seen as a boy. Her announcement echoed through our home, "I am a male". To me, this revelation was not just surprising; I approached it with a healthy dose of scepticism. Our daughter, without a history of dysphoria, had a past marked by mental health struggles.

In the ensuing days, I discovered a troubling trend within our daughter's social circle, predominantly in her drama class, where other young girls echoed similar sentiments. This peculiar movement, fuelled by the reach of social and mass media, urged young minds to believe that altering their bodies through hormones and surgeries would pave the way to a better life. A life, as I would soon find out, that was far from the truth.

I started researching as much as I could, and uncovered a narrative that I found both harmful and alarming. The message directed at young people, advocating for the reshaping of their identities, struck me as perilous. Alarmed and horrified by the accounts I found on the internet I thought, "those hormones don't belong in a body of the wrong sex. And surgery?

Cutting off healthy, integral parts of your body is an extremely drastic thing to do just because of feelings."

This apparent new trend to identify as the opposite sex struck both myself and my husband as bizarre. As we talked and tried to make sense of what was happening, we realised this situation was virtually unheard of in our circles during our youth and childhood. It seems to be a very recent phenomenon in teenage circles.

The medical profession, shockingly, seemed eager to embrace this narrative. Sophie ended up in hospital due to mental health issues, not gender dysphoria, and yet we were told that she would commit suicide if she didn't get cross-sex hormones. We resisted the immediate push to medicate our daughter and regarded the practitioner's attempts as manipulative. Like many parents in the same situation we were asked, "would you rather a live son or a dead daughter?"

We were continually met with resistance and outright rudeness from the medical professionals assigned to deal with Sophie. The urgency presented to her, coupled with the threat of her imminent demise, only deepened our scepticism.

We found it preposterous, and quite frankly, unbelievable.

As we delved into our daughter's past, we discovered a history of bullying and mental health struggles. The rush to push her into life-altering decisions seemed absurd.

Rushing a young person into a life altering decision without investigating all of the facts, the mental health history, and the underlying issues causing the gender incongruence seemed dangerous to us. We found other families online dealing with similar situations. It was confronting to realise many young girls were being rushed down this so-called 'affirmation' pathway without thoroughly analysing why.

It felt like cross-sex hormones would be something of a Band-Aid fix instead of dealing with the root cause.

Even more distressing was the fact there were so many young women regretting their decision to take testosterone and other harmful drugs.

The 'affirmation' pathway was causing irreversible harm.

Reading the stories of young people who were regretting it within a few years of embarking down this road was almost too much to bear. The hormones and the surgeries were doing more harm than good. We discovered young people's lives were being left in complete disarray. They were experiencing catastrophic harm to their bodies because they were allowed to do something which was never going to help them in the first place.

Despite our research and advocacy for our daughter, she decided to move out and to take testosterone anyway. She cut off ties with our family, leaving me and my husband and our younger son completely devastated. She moved into a shared living situation with other gender nonconforming youth but soon cried out for help after being poorly treated and finding herself suffering depression.

Sophie took testosterone for around eighteen months. In that time, her depression and other mental health issues were not alleviated. In fact, they have gotten worse.

The irreversible effects of the hormones have presented a new set of challenges—receding hairline, facial hair growth, body fat redistribution, and damage to her uterus that could lead to irreversible consequences like a hysterectomy.

The anguish the entire family has endured is beyond description. Medical practitioners have now abandoned our family. They will offer continued support for Sophie to remain on testosterone and identify as male, but they are refusing to offer services to her as a desister.

Sophie is still suffering from depression. She says she is not a girl, nor is she a boy. She won't go out or take care of herself. She doesn't eat regularly and when she does eat, it is not nutritious or healthy food. She couldn't care less about hygiene. She doesn't want anything to do with me and only allows my husband to meet her most basic needs. Her younger brother has been left confused and hurt by her behaviour.

Despite this, we are continuing to seek help for our beloved daughter.

Some medical practitioners express shock and concern, but many seem bound by a conformist silence. Fear of backlash and potential lawsuits stifle dissenting voices within the medical community, leaving parents like ourselves to navigate treacherous waters alone.

Elected politicians either ignore or refuse outright to meet with us. They remain wilfully ignorant or actively opposed to investigating the practices that have led to such horrifying consequences for our family.

I have a heart full of fierce love for my broken daughter and I refuse to be silenced.

At the time of writing this chapter, Sophie is completely estranged from us and we don't know where she is.

I am sharing my family's story and seeking to raise awareness so others can avoid living this nightmare. I have confronted politicians, embarked on letter writing campaigns, public speaking and supporting other parents in similar situations.

Strongly advocating for a Royal Commission into gender clinic practices is an important part of the way I am seeking to move forward. Other countries such as the UK, Sweden, Finland and Norway have all paused or banned medicalised 'affirmation' practices on minors after investigating the practices.

I am determined to rewrite the narrative and protect other vulnerable youth from making similar decisions that result in irreversible harm.

My daughter's life has been permanently harmed, but I am committed to ensuring that other youth can be spared the same kind of tragedy.

CHAPTER 2

Tess's story

My story begins in early 2016, which is very early to be talking about 'transgender'. At the time, most people had no idea what the term even meant, never mind believing what it was when I had the opportunity to describe it to them. Most people thought I was insane – literally.

My daughter was a much loved, much wanted, beautiful girl. She had always been petite, delicate and very 'girly'. She loved dancing, makeup, animals, mermaids, long hair and make-believe. My daughter used to play with boys mostly when she was young, because all of my friends had boys when I had her. It was a 'no brainer' to watch them play and see the differences in the sexes.

She was brought up in a home with an almost completely stay-at-home mum, and a dad that ran a small business who unfortunately wasn't able to spend heaps of time with her during the week, but was always there for her on weekends, and a grandmother who adored her. Later, we had another child to add to our family who my daughter absolutely adored. We had our usual trials, stresses and issues, but we tried our best to give her a good life.

Like many teens who end up wanting to transition, my daughter was bullied at her private school from a young age. When other concerned parents told me what they'd been seeing of the bullying, I did everything I could to try and help her. The school at the time had a very toxic environment, and even the parents of the bullies were toxic in their response to what was happening. We decided to take her out of the school in mid-primary school and put her into a local Christian school who told me they had a zero tolerance to bullying. We had tried not to run away from the problem, but after watching her at her dance lessons and seeing that she was very popular there and had no bullying issues, we decided that she wasn't the issue, and that the school environment was.

It seemed like it was a great fit for her, and for the first time in a long time, she had girl friends, and was happy. She would come out of school beaming. It was lovely to see. There's nothing parents want more than their kids to be happy and healthy.

She did well at school, she had friends, she had hobbies and she was happy.

Things started to change a couple of years into high school. Unbeknown to me at the time, a well known teacher who was her home room teacher and also took her for other subjects was an activist. He was supposedly same-sex attracted (but "not acting on it") and was actively teaching young teens in the school the ideological propaganda we now associate with programs such as Safe Schools and Respectful Relationships. To this day, I'm not sure if the school knew he was same-sex attracted or not, but I feel that they didn't because at the time, they had sacked a teacher who was in a de facto relationship as it went against their 'principles'. This teacher however was well known to be same-sex attracted in the religious community where he was also apparently a youth leader, something I found out much later. I just want to clarify, I have no issue with homosexuality, I have issues with teachers sharing their personal life experiences with young teens and the ideology that we now know is commonly taught by activist teachers.

Over a three year period, this teacher had unfettered access to these young teen minds to unfortunately twist as he saw fit. I learned that he taught them all about the use of personal pronouns, transgenderism, gay rights etc. He spoke about how Christians were terrible homophobes because they condemned gay people. He told them that it's normal for children to experiment sexually and that there was nothing wrong with it. He told them that sexually transmitted diseases were no big deal and that they just needed to go and see a doctor for treatment. He told them to go and get their own Medicare cards so that they didn't have to tell their parents.

The children in the class, who happened to be mostly boys, took these teachings literally. They were having basically sex parties at sleepovers at each other's homes and calling them 'gaming parties', so parents didn't realise. The parents obviously weren't supervising properly. My daughter used to be desperate to go to these 'gaming weekends', but I wasn't comfortable with that, so I would let her go for some evenings and pick her up afterwards.

My daughter became more secretive and would often come out with what I considered to be some unexpected statements and opinions. I thought it was just her peers' attitudes rubbing off on her; part of growing up. We would talk about these things and I thought we were pretty open and honest with each other. I knew from her telling me that she knew she could trust me and count on me (when things happened at school etc), that she meant that and that we had a good relationship.

My daughter ended up going out with one of the boys in her class when she was 14. He and his family seemed like nice people. I thought the relationship was purely platonic. They would take turns going to each other's houses on weekends or going to the movies together. My daughter used to talk to me and tell me how they were going to be married, travel the world and have a family. It was lovely to see my daughter growing up and being 'in love' for the first time.

As time went on, I started noticing times that my daughter was distressed, and I put it down to boyfriend problems. I used to ask her if she wanted to talk to me about what was going on, but she wouldn't speak to me. She had a strong stubborn streak so I knew not to push her too much.

Shortly after my daughter's 16th birthday, I knew something was wrong. She had withdrawn completely and would barely communicate with me. She was so distressed. I didn't think it was an issue with school, and I wondered whether she had broken up with her boyfriend. When I questioned her about it, she said she hadn't, but she did seem to be avoiding the issue. I tried gently to get her to talk, but she wouldn't open up. When school started, she showed no interest and was not completing her homework. She decided to stop doing her much loved dancing, something that she'd been doing since a toddler and had always been passionate about because she said she was too stressed and there was too much work to do for school. She cut off her hair, and stopped wearing her feminine clothes, opting for very casual clothes, baggy t-shirts etc. She stopped wearing makeup, wearing jewellery, etc. Her room became a complete and absolute mess. She refused to go to bed. She would be up until very late at night or early hours of the morning. She left used personal hygiene products in her room and bathroom. It was a complete change of personality. I was worried and decided to look for a psychologist to help her.

She started going to a private child psychologist in the area that was able to fit her in quickly. The appointments were expensive, but my husband and I thought it was definitely worth it if it helped her.

A few months later, late one evening after I'd returned home from being out, I went to my office and saw that my daughter had been doing her homework at my desk. She'd left a number of exercise books scattered across it. As I went to sort some papers, an exercise book opened up. It had a full page of neat writing on it; something I hadn't seen her do for a long time. I picked it up to read her work. The first line of work completely changed my life.

"It's been 7 days since *they* raped me".

I was stunned, shocked, furious, and so absolutely distraught. I felt ill, I physically wanted to be sick. I flipped through a couple more pages and it just was worse and worse. What I read was so specific in detail and so disturbing. I thought she'd been gang raped, probably the worst sort of rape there is. I somehow stumbled into her room where she was already in bed and confronted her about what happened. I was crying and asking her why she didn't tell me. I wanted her to tell me who had raped her, I couldn't understand, couldn't comprehend that this had happened. She broke down and told me the boy she was seeing had raped her while she was at his house. (The mother who was supposed to be supervising them had left them alone to go shopping for a few hours and it had happened then). I kept insisting there was someone else because of the 'they' mentioned in the book. It was then that she explained that this boy's preferred pronouns were 'they/them'. I initially thought she was covering for someone, how can they/them (plurals) be for a single person?

She ended up explaining that a specific teacher at the school had been teaching them about preferred pronouns and that many teens in her class were now referring to themselves as they/them. I asked if he'd worn a condom and she said no. I explained that we'd have to go to the doctor and get some tests done to make sure she was ok.

The next day was a Sunday, Mother's Day in fact. I'll never forget that weekend.

Monday came and I called our local police station and informed them of the rape. They made some sympathetic comments, but explained that as it had been months earlier, and the fact that they were boyfriend and girlfriend, they would not look into the rape. They didn't care that my daughter was 15 at the time, they didn't care that she was still suffering the consequences at the time. I was beyond furious. How dare the boy who'd so thoroughly destroyed my daughter be allowed to go free? I was at a complete loss as to what to do. I was scared to discuss what had happened with my husband because I didn't know how he was going to react. I didn't want to tell my ageing mother about it, and my other very close friend was the mother of the rapist, so I obviously couldn't face talking to her. I was dying inside, swinging wildly between utter rage and despair.

I was scared to even pick up my children from school in case I saw the boy. I knew he was in almost every class my daughter was in and I needed her to get away from him.

What I couldn't work out was why my daughter was still going out with him. After a long talk, I explained to her that I couldn't let her hang out with this boy on weekends any more because I was so angry that he'd hurt her so badly. She seemed to understand and accept that, despite not liking it. During this conversation, after asking why she hadn't told me earlier, she explained that she had spoken to a specific teacher at school about it and he'd told her that she needed to chalk the rape up to life experience and that the boy loved her and so she needed to forgive him. Looking through her diary further, she'd actually written about talking to the teacher. She'd written that she couldn't stand the boy touching her in any way, but was working to forgive him. I decided on a plan.

We needed a new therapist for our daughter. It was obvious that the therapist my daughter had been seeing hadn't been helping, because I was convinced that if she had been, she would have already worked out the reason behind my daughter's distress. I called around other therapists, looking for someone who wouldn't cut me out of the process. I wanted to be able to talk to them about what had been happening and would communicate with me.

We needed to get her away from this boy and being that he was in every class with her, we needed to get her out of the school. She was hating school and not doing well, except for one TAFE class that she did there, so I investigated to see whether she could just do the course at TAFE full time. I thought that if TAFE was a possibility, it would be a good way for her to leave the school, open her horizons and meet some other people. This would hopefully lead to her breaking up with this boy.

It took about a month to get into TAFE as a minor, and I contacted the school to let them know what had happened and why we were pulling her out immediately. The lady on the phone was a little shocked at my revelations, but was more concerned about the fact that I refused to pay a term's fees upfront to exit the school. I expected her to let the principal know what had happened, but I learned later that that never eventuated.

The more I read through the diary, the more I found that the teacher was a very disturbed person. He had been actively encouraging the teens in the class to experiment sexually and then come back to class and discuss it. This was why my daughter had been so upset periodically, because the boy she'd been dating was going to these sex parties on weekends and having sex with other boys and she was insanely jealous about it. Her journal entries talked about how she thought her thoughts were wrong and she needed to work on feeling jealous. Her journal also explained that she'd spoken to the teacher about her feelings and he confirmed that what the boys were doing was normal and natural and her feelings were wrong. How could my daughter be so confused? I tried and tried to reason with her that she wasn't in a healthy relationship, that if he respected her and cared for her, he wouldn't have raped her and he wouldn't be having sex with others. Unfortunately, she was so brainwashed she just didn't seem to understand why it was a problem.

I was able to find a therapist who was more parent centred and I had an appointment with her before she met my daughter. I took the diary along as this therapist was an expert in testifying in court about sexual assaults etc, so I thought it would be good for her to see it and get her opinion on whether it would be good evidence, and to see if she had any ideas on how we could proceed forward with getting my daughter some justice. The therapist was saddened reading parts of the journal and very concerned about the teens and especially the teacher. I had high hopes that she would be able to help my daughter with her trauma. The combination of starting TAFE and getting decent therapy really started to make a visible difference in my daughter's behaviour and attitude. She would have issues with anxiety, but we seemed to be working through it. About a month after she started TAFE, the boy she'd been seeing broke up with her. She was completely heartbroken, but I was so relieved!

I kept contacting different branches of the police to see if we could get anyone to press charges against the boy, but no one was interested in the case. I wasn't sure how to handle the issue of the teacher at school either. The rape hadn't happened at school, but the teacher was definitely grooming the teens and teaching them things that should not be taught in a religious school. I was so traumatised myself; I was struggling to cope with everything. I didn't want to traumatise my daughter further by being dragged into school to be questioned, but I didn't want to let it go either. If the police weren't interested, why would the school be? The decision was sort of taken out of my hands when my daughter advised me that he'd left Australia and was working in a school in Canada. Unbeknownst to me at the time, this man was friends with his students on Facebook. My daughter had advised him that I'd learned of the rape and he'd fled the country, no doubt knowing he'd be in trouble as he hadn't reported the rape of a minor.

At this point, my daughter had decided to start telling some of her friends what had happened and why she'd left the school so unexpectedly. They mostly didn't believe her. The boy in question appeared very friendly and charming, and they all sided with him. The only friend she still had was one boy in the class who was not friends with the rapist. Strangely, the family used to be friends but something had happened that had broken up the two families completely. I didn't have a clue as to why at the time. (I much later found out that it was because the rapist had also attempted to rape this boy too and he'd been quite traumatised by it). They became quite close and I was happy as at least she still had one peer who believed her. I had worked with this boy's mother briefly and although I wouldn't have called her anything more than a casual acquaintance, it did give me a bit of comfort knowing that we had mutual friends so she must be an OK person.

One day my daughter told me that this boy had decided he was a girl and had changed his name to a female name. She told me she thought it was really weird but he was a nice boy who'd stuck by her so she wasn't going to judge. I thought it was totally bizarre that this boy (whose mother I knew and had worked with, who had played sports etc as a child and seemed like a normal boy) thought he was a girl. I wasn't sure what to say in response to this revelation. I suggested that she avoid using the female name as much as possible and to try and get him to speak to his mum. The school he attended was still calling him by his birth name so she should too.

A while later, my daughter suddenly announced that she was a lesbian. I was very surprised as she'd always liked boys and had used to point them out to me and talk about them etc. My thoughts immediately went to wondering if this was in response to the rape trauma, as she'd still been experiencing depression and anxiety. After asking her if she had met someone she liked or if it was more of a general feeling, I was very confused when she told me she was in love with the boy who wanted to be known by the girl's name. I wasn't sure how to respond to this, so I thought I'd go with the truth. I told her that I understood this boy was wanting to be a girl and using a new female name, but he was still a boy and so she wasn't what would be considered a lesbian, but straight.

What happened next shocked me completely. My daughter had a complete meltdown. I'd never seen anything like it. I was told that I didn't know the new biology, that old biology was wrong and that you could change sex. That I didn't know what I was talking about (despite lots of study of anatomy and the human body). For a moment, I stood there completely stunned – had I missed something? What was happening that someone could think you could suddenly change sex? I calmly tried to talk about chromosomes and how they worked in the body but she just got more and more upset until she stormed out. I started some serious investigation about changing sex, which led me to the term transgender and I started to read everything I could lay my hands on.

I read about Alfred Kinsey and John Money and the experiments that they'd done. It sickened me. I wanted to print out everything I'd found as I went deeper and deeper into this rabbit hole, but I was terrified my daughter would find what I was looking at, so I copied the URL's of the articles and saved them on a document I renamed and hid. This search eventually led me to Victoria's resources on Safe Schools. I looked at Minus 18, and was even more horrified to see links to places where you could buy small size condoms and how to make sex toys from simple home gadgets such as electric toothbrushes. The more I read, the more sickened I became as I quickly figured out this was what the groomer teacher had been teaching my daughter and the others in his classes. Most infuriating was a document I'd found on the Minus 18 Website, explaining in detail about how to hide browser history from parents on all the different operating systems. How could an organisation like this that an education department was promoting freely give children this information? I was the mother who'd gone to all the cyber safety and security talks that took place at school, I was strict with screen time and what my children were allowed to see and do. I felt like a schmuck.

A good friend of mine sent me a video of a mother in a different state talking about the sexualised content her children had come home from school and described to her. I couldn't believe what I was hearing. This was exactly what I'd found already online. I joined her Facebook group and began talking to other mums there who were discussing similar, very disturbing content in schools. I met one Victorian mother whose 12 year old son had been shown an anal sex video in his year seven classroom at a Victorian school and he'd been so shocked and disgusted that he'd developed cardiac symptoms which had been diagnosed as PTSD. She talked about how her son had completely changed personality and how they were struggling to get him to 'function' normally again. It was so similar in so many ways to my daughter's trauma story, that we became fast friends. Finally I had someone to talk to that didn't think I was insane.

A few weeks later, my daughter announced that she was in fact a boy. She'd always been a boy, but she'd been born in the wrong body. I was so confused. I asked her why she would think that. She had always been so happily feminine up until the rape. She was already menstruating, had a female figure with curvy hips, and breasts. She tried to explain that gender has nothing to do with biological sex which I thought was ludicrous at the time. My thoughts on this were very 'science based'. I knew people were sometimes born with both sets of sex organs, (intersex), but I knew this was not the case with my daughter so I couldn't comprehend what she meant.

I took her to see our family doctor who after talking to us together and then to her alone, referred us to the gender clinic at the children's hospital. In my state of shock and ignorance I was quite pleased that we were going to see experts to sort this out. I assumed that they would talk to her, do thorough examinations and then tell her that she was completely female. It was going to take months of waiting to get in so in the meantime we kept seeing her psychologist. I was furious that the doctor started calling her by a new name. Nothing had been decided so how dare they just decide to go along with this obvious delusion? They were supposed to have studied the human body. Human beings don't change sex. I wrote to the doctor later and expressed my disgust.

What I didn't understand at the time was that the therapist had seen her cut her hair and wearing baggy clothes as confirmation that she was indeed a male trapped in a female body, and had simply been affirming her. No science was required for this ideology. What my daughter said went. It was recommended to us that we use her new preferred name and gender (which I refused to do), and that we remove all photos, and anything else that would remind her of her 'former life' as a girl. I refused to do this also. Of course, she'd always been a girl so suddenly turning my back on my memories was unacceptable to me.

At this point I felt as if I was living a dual existence. While not affirming my daughter, I was trying to be the peacekeeper and not show my pain and my fear for my daughter. With my research I began to look up things like 'my daughter suddenly thinks she's a male', I found an article by a website called 4th Wave Now. This was a turning point for me. It described a phenomenon called Rapid Onset Gender Dysphoria ("ROGD"). It was the first time I'd heard of the term and I was ecstatic! It all made perfect sense. It was exactly what my daughter was going through. I remember sitting in my bed crying in relief that someone understood what was happening. Now I had a term to research, I spent hours researching the phenomenon and found that parents all over the world were experiencing this sudden and complete change of personality with their children. I found myself going for drives and parking at parks to make phone calls to people and organisations about the issue as I was terrified my daughter might find out that I did not agree with what she was doing.

My Victorian friend, with some long distance help from me, organised a protest against what was known at the time as 'Safe Schools' (an oxymoron if ever I heard one). This process showed us very early on just what we were up against. We couldn't believe the fear many people showed when asked to stand up to defend the innocence of our children. Very few people thought we would succeed. We were mocked by many for even trying. Our social media pages, groups and profiles were shut down while talking about the protest, and we were not able to advertise the event at all. With the help of a small number of individuals, we did hold a successful protest. It was a first of its kind. While it didn't stop anything from continuing, it did help us to connect with many people we would not have ordinarily come into contact with, and it gave us experience and showed us who we could trust.

I had spoken to my daughter about what I was doing trying to stop the sexualisation of young children. I showed her activity sheets that I'd found while doing my research and she too understood that children were too young to learn these topics.

Another turning point for me was discovering the website, Parents of ROGD Kids. After browsing their website, I contacted them and poured out my heart about what had been happening. A short time later, they responded with a link to a survey that had been written to support Lisa Littman's study into the ROGD phenomena. To say it was comprehensive was an understatement. It took me a good couple of hours to complete. I felt it was definitely worth my time to participate in this study if it would help even a single person.

Daily life was a struggle. I was working and would get calls from my daughter at TAFE saying she was having a panic attack and needed me to come and collect her. Fortunately I was in a position with my work to be able to do so without too much grief. The thing that confused me though is that when I collected her, she was her normal self. She'd want to go shopping, or show me some place 'cool' during her time in the city. While I was happy to do this and connect with her, I wondered why she thought she was having panic attacks as there was literally no trace of them. Anxiety is unfortunately something I know too well personally, and what she was experiencing just didn't fit the picture.

I was trying desperately to keep things 'normal' for everyone in the family. I was spending as much time as I could with my daughter trying to show that I loved and supported her. I was working, being a wife and mother and I also had a younger child that needed a great deal of attention due to medical issues. Every spare moment, I was trying to research, to find a solution, to get all the information I could to help my daughter and to make sense of the information I was learning.

At about 3 am one morning, my younger child came and woke me and told me that my daughter had friends in her room and that she'd woken him up. Startled and confused, I went to her room and found my daughter in her room with her laptop and phone still dressed in her clothes from the day before, having shown absolutely no signs of having even been asleep.

I'd been that mum who'd gone to all the cyber safety classes the school had run. We had strict rules about devices in bedrooms. At night they were all supposed to be plugged in and charging on our kitchen bench, ready for school the next day. Not only had she woken her sibling and also myself, but it was 3am and she needed to be up at 6am to go to TAFE. She was immediately remorseful and hung up her phone while I told her off for breaking the rules and having her devices in her room. It dawned on me that the panic attacks she'd been having at TAFE were more likely that she had been tired from staying up talking to friends all night. I took her devices and told her if I caught her doing this again, she'd lose her device privileges.

The next day I talked to her and we discussed that she wasn't giving herself a chance to heal and feel better with her anxiety and depression by not getting enough sleep. I explained that the repeated calls for me to stop work and collect her was causing issues with my work too. She said all the right things to make me feel she'd understood and that she wouldn't do it again.

The very same evening at around 3 am again, I was woken by my younger child and told that my daughter had woken him again. I jumped out of bed and surprised her by going into her room and finding her in just her underwear, taking topless photos of herself while talking to a group of her friends on her laptop. I saw red. I was beyond furious! I grabbed the phone from her and saw that she'd shared the photos to her friends and that they'd responded with comments about how masculine she looked. If I hadn't been so furious, I would have laughed! Here was my beautiful daughter in just her underwear showing her breasts and her lovely feminine curves, and someone was telling her she looked masculine?

We'd talked extensively about sharing intimate photos over the internet, and it had been an issue when I'd found out about her being raped, and here she was doing it again? Unbelievable!

She was very upset that I'd again caught her. I told her she'd lost her device privileges so she could have her phone and laptop for TAFE, but she wouldn't have access at home for two weeks. At this point we still had a landline and I explained that she could still call her friends and talk that way. I reminded her that just that day she'd blatantly lied to me and told me that she wouldn't do it again.

A couple of days later, in early December, my whole life changed.

After a knock on the door which my daughter answered, she led in a young person, well dressed in a suit. This person looked remarkably like one of her group of friends and I incorrectly assumed it was him, all dressed up for some reason. My daughter and this person stood awkwardly looking at me. I asked what this person was doing here, and the person calmly replied that my son was in danger and that he was here to take him away.

I immediately stood up, and asked what he meant. How was my son in danger? He told me that my son was in emotional danger and that he had to leave immediately.

What on earth?

Emotional danger? I asked him again for his name and where he was from. He responded rudely that he'd already told me who he was and that he was from a trans activist organisation. When he said this, I worked out that he was not there to take my actual son, but my daughter! I asked him for identification, a court order, anything, that might give him the authority to come into my home and try to take my minor child. He kept speaking to me as if I was a complete idiot and was extremely arrogant and self-assured that he had every right to be in my house and take my daughter!

I told him to leave the house and he refused. I repeated the request several times and he ended up pushing past me and following my daughter into her room where they began throwing together some of her things into a bag. I asked my elderly mother who was with me to call 000. She did and handed me the phone.

I told the police what was happening. I told them that there was a man in the house with no identification trying to take my daughter and that I needed help urgently. The operator asked how old my daughter was and they told me that at age 16, if she wanted to go with him, I couldn't stop her!!!!

Imagine my feelings of complete helplessness at that point. I was absolutely stunned, in shock, and shaking. I was trying to grab the items they were putting into a bag and he kept stopping me. In the end he pushed past me and I managed to get between him and my daughter and as he was walking through the front door with her belongings, I managed to literally push him out of the door while my mum was pulling my daughter away from the door and I managed to lock it. The man was bashing at the door and threatening to call the police. My daughter was trying to get out. I ended up key locking all the doors and windows as I was terrified and then called my husband at work and told him to get home immediately as I needed help.

I was hysterical. Shaking, dry reaching, screaming. My poor younger son and my mum stood there watching everything that was happening with very shocked expressions. I was scared that my poor mother would have a heart attack or another stroke. My daughter just looked on blankly. I didn't know what to do. If the police weren't going to help me, who would?

In the meantime, as the activist had tripped after I'd pushed him through my front door, he'd called the police and they'd come for him. I was standing looking out a window to the front of my house and I watched as the police came and spoke to this activist. I was enraged! What a slap in the face that they wouldn't come for me, but they'd come to help this revolving activist who was trying to take my child! I felt as if I was having an out-of-world experience, a living nightmare; that I was stuck in the Twilight Zone. How dare the police not help me, when an intruder had been in my house, trying to take my child, who knows where, when I was her mother who loved her?

They knocked on the front door and I opened it. They asked to come in. I refused. I was not going to talk to the police when they were so obviously not here to help me. I told them to get lost and not to come back and to get the activist off my property and away from my family.

My husband came home and as he pulled up the police went and spoke to him. I hadn't told my husband what was happening, and being a good, law-abiding citizen, when the police asked if they could come in and talk, he let them in. I was so angry that they were in my house. I felt like they were the enemy and they were playing along with this activist and putting us at risk. I was inconsolable. I calmed down enough to tell them what had happened. They asked to speak to my daughter who had slunk away to her room as she obviously couldn't face me. The police asked her for her version of events and she proceeded to tell them that she did not feel safe. I couldn't believe what she was saying! How could she not feel safe in a home where the whole world was revolving around trying to support her? They asked what she meant and this is where I heard the very obvious scripting that people had been writing about in articles.

A parent knows how their child speaks. The words they use, the sentence structure. My daughter suddenly changed before my eyes as if she were acting a role. She used words that she likely didn't even understand and were definitely not in her normal vocabulary. Her sentence structure changed completely too. As I listened to her speak, I kept saying to the police, 'ask her what that word means, I bet she doesn't know'. She told them she didn't feel safe emotionally. They told her that the activist outside had told them that she was suicidal. She agreed that she was. Again, a total surprise for me. She'd been going to the psychologist weekly and even the psychologist had reported that she was doing really well. The police questioned her about how she thought she might suicide and she was unable to give them an answer. The police suggested it was more of a feeling than an actual thing she was going to do and she agreed with them.

The police explained that as she said she was suicidal they had to take her into custody for a psychiatric evaluation. I had absolutely no issue with this at all. I didn't think she was suicidal, but welcomed another opinion.

While she went to get something from her room, the officers said that they didn't think she was genuinely suicidal and were very apologetic. The police explained that they were taking her to the local hospital and that we were welcome to follow and wait, but we'd be in a different area.

My husband and I waited in the waiting room for hours. Me, mostly quietly crying, still shaking and very much in shock, and my daughter in another area with the two police officers for company. We were taken into an office by the hospital social worker who affirmed that we were indeed terrible parents because we were deadnaming (what transgender activists call using someone's birth name) and misgendering her. I tried to explain that I refused to give in to my daughter's delusion because we hadn't even gone to see the experts at the gender clinic yet. They couldn't understand why I took this stance because as far as the social worker was concerned, the fact that my daughter had announced that she was trans, meant that she *was*. We were told that that child is dead to us now, we have a son… "better a live son, than a dead daughter". A line that was repeated to us and to every parent facing this challenge repeatedly.

I didn't understand how the social worker could say this. When I had first started reading about the transgender issue, it immediately made me think of a person with anorexia nervosa. I'd had two cousins go through this in their teens and I'd spent a lot of time with one specifically and I saw how emaciated she was and how much she genuinely believed that she was fat. I saw how depressed she'd been and how determined she was to lose weight and I'd been there at least once for a suicide attempt and had seen how desperately devastated she was.

I explained this to the social worker. How is it that we were expected to go along with my daughter's very unhealthy delusion (because every delusion is unhealthy surely), and suddenly start acting as if she's something she's not and will never be? The social worker was rude, treated us like we were absolute dirt, showed no compassion or empathy and told us that we were bigots and transphobic. How dare we compare transgender to anorexia!

During the time waiting with the police officers in another part of the hospital, my daughter had spoken to them about her rape. The police officers came and spoke to me in the waiting room about it, wanting to know all the details. I willingly gave them all the details of everything that I knew had happened and the details I'd read about in the diary. I explained that I still had the diary as evidence as I was hoping to find someone who was willing to investigate and finally bring some justice to my daughter.

The police asked if I would go home and get the diary and give it to them as they seemed keen to investigate. I was so happy and relieved that finally someone was taking the rape seriously. I gave them the rapists' name, contact details, parent details etc and they promised to investigate. After we returned back to the hospital with the diary, as I went to hand it over, I felt as if a bolt of lightning had hit me. I was suddenly questioning whether I should actually hand it over given I didn't have a copy of it. The police held one side, while I held the other side, not letting go. I looked up at the police officer and asked did he promise I would get it back? He assured me I definitely would have it returned. He explained that I had the incident number and the evidence receipt and that while he made no promises, he would investigate and that they would then return it to me. I cautiously handed it over.

Finally the psychiatrist came and said that he'd done an evaluation and that my daughter was not suicidal. He basically suggested that she was being a difficult teen. He said he doubted the transgender part was anything serious, but just to go along with her wishes anyway. He said he had no problem in allowing us to take her home, but said that we should use her new name and pronouns. Another social worker had come on duty by that time and we were called in and told again that we had to respect our daughter's wishes and that even though our daughter had been cleared of being suicidal that she would become so if we didn't go along with her wishes. Again, 'better a live son than a dead daughter'. Our daughter had agreed to come home with us but we were not allowed to punish her for anything, we were not allowed to take away any of her devices, or limit her time on them in any way. We were not allowed to stop her from going out, limit her bed time or basically parent her in any way.

I was completely mentally, physically and emotionally destroyed. I came home and had to explain everything that had been happening to my mother. I had decided not to burden her with the rape or the transgender announcement, I wanted to spare her the heartache and the devastation that we'd been going through.

That evening, I had a call from the head of the trans organisation, who apologised for what had occurred. He agreed that the activist should not have come to our home. I asked if there would be some sort of punishment or expulsion from the group but he said no. He was able to explain that my daughter had called her boyfriend who was transitioning and told him that I'd banned her from having her devices at home for 2 weeks. He'd told his mother (who had fully accepted that her son was now female and put him onto puberty blockers immediately). The mum was horrified that I was so abusive and was putting my daughter into such danger, that she called the activist and together made the plan to rescue her from her terrible, horrible, abusive home situation. I was in such a world of isolation and stress. I couldn't sleep. I was terrified that the activist would come back and try to take our daughter again, or that my daughter would try to run away. I lay in bed with the house keys in my hand, listening to every little noise. I would get up, creep through the house and make sure everything was ok, before returning to bed and laying awake, trying not to let my guard slip. My mother would come to my house during the day and I would give her the keys and ask her to keep watch over everything while I tried to sleep. If I did happen to doze, I had nightmares about trans activists forcing their way into my house and taking my children. We had a call from a person from the hospital saying they were sending someone to our house to talk to us. I was scared to let anyone into the house or to talk to anyone, but wanted to make sure we were doing the right thing for our daughter and our family.

The woman who came was not on our side. She reminded me of a toad, sitting cross legged in one of our armchairs, blurting out how wrong we were about everything on every level. She interrogated my husband and I for around seven hours. She looked at the pigsty that was my daughter's room and told us how terrible we were for having photos of my daughter as a toddler proudly displayed around the house. We were told how terrible we were that my daughter's room had not been repainted. We had been slowly painting room by room but had not reached her room yet.

My daughter's room was not a normal level of mess. It was literally almost knee high filled with garbage of all sorts and it stank. Despite being told not to, she left food in her room along with used sanitary products, dirty clothes, pieces of paper, and lolly wrappers. I would go through with a garbage bag to try and gain control, but it would lead to her getting so angry with me. We were in the midst of a stalemate. I asked the therapist how I could even access her room to paint it, but she couldn't answer. The woman told us we should ask my daughter to clean it as it was her responsibility (as if we hadn't tried that!). The whole day was a waste of time, only allowing me to feel like Alice in Wonderland who'd fallen down a rabbit hole and was dealing with the Mad Hatter and his crazy friends.

Her parting words again were that we were transphobic, we had to let our daughter lead our household with her wants and demands. We immediately had to repaint her room, take down the baby photos and never refer to our daughter as a daughter again. 'Better a live son, than a dead daughter'. We decided not to do anything different until we'd been to the gender clinic.

The hospital had given me a phone number for an organisation called PFLAG (Parents and Friends of Lesbian and Gays). I phoned them in tears and told them what had been happening. The person on the phone was sympathetic and understood the term transgender but the sympathy stopped when I asked if they knew someone who could actually help my daughter come out of this delusion. The woman questioned why I wouldn't celebrate my 'son' becoming her true, authentic self.

I contacted a well known parenting expert, who I'd gone and listened to a year earlier, but I had an email response with a PFLAG number and some other crisis line numbers. I contacted family organisations and even religious organisations who were at least helpful in that they listened to me without telling me I was abusive, but they were no help either. I contacted Parents of ROGD Kids again to see if they knew anyone who could help.

I was so traumatised, I barely functioned. I used to go out to a local park at night and cry so I didn't upset my family. I was so traumatised, I didn't know what to do. I was scared of being in the house alone. I was scared to leave the house. I couldn't go to work. I was diagnosed with PTSD and as a result, I stopped being able to talk to people on the phone. I started having trouble with my speech, not being able to say the words I wanted to say. I stopped being able to go to our local shop as I was scared to see the other people involved. I cried all the time. I lost interest in everything. I lost friendships because people were either too scared to see me as I wasn't coping or they disagreed with me and thought I should have celebrated my once perfectly normal daughter 'coming out'.

We were told at the hospital that my daughter was to attend the local CAMHS (Child and Adolescent Mental Health Service) as my daughter didn't want to see her psychologist any more.

The CAMHS appointment was also traumatic for me. It was obvious from the minute we got there that they were going to immediately affirm. The psychologist she was allocated would barely speak to me, dismissing all my comments and concerns. After a few weeks, he called me in and told me he didn't think that my daughter was a genuine case. That he was focussing on trying to get her to be a functioning member of society and dealing with the rape trauma which would allow her to venture out more etc. I was pretty happy about that. At least he wasn't pushing her. However, I found out from my daughter much later that he'd actually been lying to me. This therapist had told my daughter all my concerns and was also helping her to get away from us.

Some time later, I received a response from Parents of ROGD Kids. They were sympathetic, and told me they were receiving so many calls for help, they asked if I would consider starting a support group for parents. They explained that they'd been getting lots of requests for help from parents in Australia and New Zealand and they thought since I'd done so much research and was actively trying to make people understand the harms of what the early comprehensive sexualisation programs were doing to our teens, that I'd be a good candidate for a group leader. I immediately said yes! Maybe this was the answer. I could connect with other parents who were feeling scared and lost like me, and we could at least talk freely without being told we were crazy or abusive.

It was super difficult to start with. I was struggling with my speech and weird fear of the phone, but I decided I could either fall into more of a heap, or push myself to do it. I chose to push.

The first contact they gave me was on the other side of the country, but we connected and were able to commiserate together. I was getting a number of contacts each week. It was sad, but so wonderful to have other parents from different parts of the country that I was able to connect with and receive support from.

During these conversations I was learning a great deal too. Although our children were different ages, different backgrounds, and living in different parts of the country, the actions the children took, the way they made their announcements etc were remarkably similar. They all used the same terminology and even expressed the same thoughts. More and more I was noticing that these children and teens had either experienced significant trauma, were autistic or had some other sort of diagnosis of a personality disorder. More worrying was that the medical professionals' responses to these situations were all the same too. All the parents who expressed doubts about the immediate affirmation of a child's new persona, were all 'abusive', 'bigots', 'transphobic'. Medical professionals seemed comfortable hiding information from parents, lying by omission and actively participating in doing just what the parents had expressed they didn't want, behind their backs. All the parents were scared to talk to strangers, despite everything being vetted. Some parents didn't want to talk about their situations at all, until they'd heard my situation. My opening up and making myself vulnerable seemed to get them to trust me. All the parents were the same; they just wanted me to wave around a magic wand and make things better for them.

I started feeling more and more responsible to these parents so I went to talks about this topic and would talk to the people talking at the event, hoping they knew something that would help. Back in 2016, if you went and started talking to people about transitioning, they mostly thought you were insane. Of course you can't change sex, who's crazy enough to think you can? It took a great deal of convincing to get anyone to believe you, even 'experts'. It was so difficult, but I kept pushing and pushing myself to try and get help. Hearing parents' stories and living with the day-to-day difficulties we were experiencing made me more and more determined. I was on a roller coaster of emotions, sometimes experiencing such deep despair that I could barely bring myself to get out of bed, sometimes the rage was so all consuming that I couldn't stop moving for fear I'd explode. I'd use this rage and get onto my computer and research and write letters and emails to everyone I could think of.

We received an appointment for the youth gender clinic at the beginning of the new year. The letter referred to my daughter as my son, and used her new name. I couldn't understand this. I had previously worked in a hospital. Hospitals used official names, names on Medicare cards, not nicknames and preferred names and pronouns. I called to confirm the appointment and asked why the letter used the wrong name. My daughter hadn't officially changed her name. They explained that they used the new preferred name to respect the patient, however, the letter was addressed to me, so how would that offend my daughter?

The day of the appointment came. My daughter was excited. I was hopeful that we'd get some help. The first appointment was an introductory appointment with the clinic nurse, Amanda, who would explain how the gender clinic worked. I expected some time to talk to the nurse without my daughter being present, however that was not the case at all. We were directed to sit down in an interview room together with Amanda, calling my daughter my son and using the wrong name every single time. At times it was as if Amanda was using the wrong name more than necessary, just to rub it in.

Amanda handed my daughter what I later learned was a consent form. It looked like a worksheet that someone might give a year 6 child at school. Amanda talked about the side effects of taking puberty blockers and cross sex hormones in the most stupidly simplistic way. Things like, 'your red blood cell count might go up a little, but all you need to do is donate blood each month, and you'll be fine…" My daughter at that point dutifully scribbled a note on that point saying 'donate blood every month'. No mention of the damage to the liver that is possible with increased red blood cell count, no mention of the increased risk of cancer, nothing of the serious side effects like sterility, loss of cognitive function amongst other issues I'd read about. As the seconds ticked by in that room, I felt as if blow after blow was landing on my chest. I felt ill.

The conversation between Amanda and my daughter stopped suddenly and Amanda looked at me and asked what I felt about starting my 'son' on puberty blockers straight away. WHAT?????? How was I going to answer this, with my daughter sitting next to me and me desperately wanting to keep her onside? I was literally breaking into a sweat, when I think I was hit by some divine intervention.

I told Amanda that since my daughter had been a few months old, I'd been using natural medicine to help her as she'd had many ear infections as a child. I told Amanda my journey with my daughter had led me to a very natural lifestyle where I cooked from scratch, and used very little medicine. I told her that I was absolutely uncomfortable with polluting her body with artificial medications that carried side effects. I thought this was a great non-confrontational answer. I was also extremely confused as to why we were being offered puberty blockers before we'd even seen the professionals. I told Amanda that I was confused as to why we were being offered puberty blockers, when my daughter was obviously past initial puberty. She'd just turned 17 at this point. Amanda looked at me and said that perhaps she should skip puberty blockers and go into cross sex hormones. Again WHAT????? How was it possible that we were being offered these drugs within the first 25 minute appointment before we'd even seen the specialists? I responded again that I wasn't comfortable with chemical medications. Amanda asked how my husband felt about it, and I told her he thought the same as me. Without skipping a beat, Amanda told my daughter that given her age, it would take too long to go through a court process so she'd have to wait until she turned 18 to start drug therapy. My daughter was absolutely livid with me and things were very uncomfortable for weeks. Our next appointment at the gender clinic was with the psychiatrist and psychologist. We were again seated in an office together being asked a million questions. My daughter and I were then separated and interviewed. I held nothing back in that conversation, openly expressing my concerns and confusion. I talked about the complete change of personality my daughter had gone through after the rape, and how she'd not had real trauma counselling, how instead the therapy had been solely focused on transitioning. The psychiatrist told me that rape trauma had absolutely nothing to do with gender dysphoria and that my daughter had always been a male trapped in a female body. Again, I tried to use the anorexia analogy, only to be shot down and told that gender dysphoria was not a mental condition. I was furious and in complete disbelief. I couldn't believe this so-called professional was completely denying biology.

My daughter and I were brought together again and told that at the next appointment she would see the endocrinologist who would measure and take photographs so they could keep track of the changes that would occur with her body after she started hormones.

I had expected the gender clinic would take blood tests, check her hormone levels and make sure everything was normal. I expected them to take the rape trauma seriously and tell her she needed extensive counselling to bring her back to a semblance of the fun loving, feminine person she'd been. I was shocked that the only counselling they were concerned with was how to assimilate in society as this new fake persona.

I did not attend another session at the gender clinic with my daughter, because 9 months after the activist came to our home to try and take my daughter, she disappeared one night while we were out. She took the bare minimum, and left a note saying that until we acknowledged her as our son and that I'd given birth to two sons, she would not speak to me. We called the police as we were concerned. I didn't think she had any money, she'd left her medication at home and I was concerned about her safety. The police did find her. She was staying at the activist's house. They wouldn't bring her back or tell us where she was though. I contacted the head of the trans organisation and he replied that he was happy she'd escaped such an abusive situation.

I was obviously devastated, but in the coming days there was also a profound sense of relief. I felt as if I could breathe for the first time in a long time. No more tip toeing around her constant demands. No more avoiding calling her by her name, no more worrying about people breaking into the house and taking her. I missed her with every fibre of my being, and I was terrified for her, but I was also free to be me. I could take calls from people without worrying about her listening in to conversations, I could print out articles and emails and not be scared of her finding them.

The only other fear that remained was that because I'd been labelled abusive, I was on constant alert that someone would come and try to take custody of my son. We wrapped him up in cotton wool to protect him from the world. He was not allowed to answer the door, he was not allowed to speak to anyone about what had been happening or what I was doing. We taught him that if the police or anyone ever came to school and asked for him, that he was to leave the school immediately and to go to our office which was a short walk away. Why is it that if as a parent, you're considered abusive, does the state not come after the remaining siblings and try and take them to safety???

I got a call from Centrelink (our national social security scheme) who initially asked me if I was the mother of "new name". They got me on a particularly bad day of the grief rollercoaster and I was furious that they were an official government body and called me using an assumed name. I said no I wasn't. The woman on the phone asked me a few different ways about this male child with a specific name. Eventually she broke down and said my daughter's name. I told her yes I was. The woman asked me why my daughter wasn't able to live at home. Stunned, I told her that I'd never kicked her out and that she had her room here at home as she'd left it. The woman told me my daughter had applied for extra funding for being away from home and so she needed to know if she was still welcome. I told her that I loved my daughter and that she was always welcome at her home. I questioned the woman about how my daughter had managed to get a new name and gender on a new Medicare card while being under 18 and not legally changing her name, and was told that the government offices had been told that if anyone says they're trans, they have to use whatever name and gender they are told regardless of what any other identification has to say. This means that people can now have multiple Medicare cards. So, despite the fact that she was still a minor, and was still on our Medicare Card with her birth name, she also had another Medicare Card with her new assumed (not legal name) and not only that, we were not allowed to remove her! My daughter had used the card to open a bank account and have payments from Centrelink to stay away from home.

Throughout this time, it was ironic that the only 'right' we seem to have (according to the Education Department who contacted us every couple of weeks or so after we pulled her out of school, and put her into full time TAFE,) is to be legally liable if our children don't attend school, regardless of whether we even know where they are! Despite having given my daughter's TAFE admission paperwork to her high 2school, proving she was enrolled at TAFE as a minor, the school had reported us to the Education Department for withdrawing her from the school system. As she had stopped attending TAFE when she ran away, we were constantly threatened with having charges brought against us by the Education Department. Eventually I gave the woman at the Education Department the police officer's name that had contacted us with her location and told her to take it up with him. The phone calls were constantly like rubbing salt into the wound of my grief.

Since early in the year, we had also tried to contact the police officers who had promised to investigate the rape, but they never responded to emails or voice messages. Now that we were free to do more without my daughter being in the middle and risk getting her off-side, we decided to chase up the diary. I was furious at the school for allowing a groomer teacher into its midst. I wanted the teacher punished too and that diary was the only evidence I had.

My husband decided to go to the police station to get the diary back. He spoke with the officers at the station, and when he returned home, he looked very grey, like he was about to pass out. I asked him what was wrong and he proceeded to tell me the police had destroyed the diary!

I couldn't believe what he was telling me! How could the police destroy evidence into the rape of a minor (remember, my daughter had been 15 at the time)? A wave of emotions coursed through me that I just couldn't control. I started sobbing. How could they? I raced out of the office we were in and marched to the police station, sobbing hysterically the whole way, my poor husband trying to keep up behind me. I was terrified that he'd try to stop me, and I kept screaming at him to leave me alone. I was way past being rational, I wanted to scream and rage. I was so completely and utterly broken and devastated.

Inside the police station, people were milling around and I pushed past everyone, screaming and telling everyone I wanted to speak to whoever was in charge. A kind officer at the desk told me the evidence had been destroyed and she couldn't give me the answers as to why as the police officer who'd made the decision was in another local branch. She drew me a map of where to go and I left, again with my husband trailing behind me. I was still sobbing, screaming sometimes. I felt like I was having a breakdown. I stopped traffic and pushed past a police officer on horseback in my determination to see this officer who'd destroyed our chance for justice. I'm embarrassed now to think about what a spectacle I made of myself, but at the time, I was barely functioning.

Arriving at the building, there was no reception so I pressed the attendance button and screamed to open the door. After waiting a couple of minutes, I remembered that on my way there, just around the corner, was our police minister's office. I decided I would go and talk to them there.

In the meantime, my husband waited at the office door for the police officer. They arrived shortly after I'd walked away and my husband had told them the situation and that I was hysterical and wanting their heads on a platter. The Detective Sergeant saw this as a threat and called for backup.

In the Police Minister's office, the staff there were trying to calm me down. They gave me tissues and water while I blurted out my story. Unfortunately the minister was not there at the time so I was unable to talk to her. A call from my husband asking where I was made me head out, but not before leaving my details with the staff for the minister to contact me as I'd told them I wanted to make a formal complaint.

Having calmed down a fraction, I made my way back to the Police office where I was met with the Detective Sergeant, in plain clothes, and a fully armed police officer with gun and taser and vest. I actually laughed! I figured out that my husband had told them about my state and the officer had been scared to see me without backup.

We were led up to an office, similar to what is seen in crime shows with a desk and some chairs. We sat down and between the hysterical hiccups and tears, I told them the story of what had happened, trying to keep calm. The Detective Sergeant reached over and touched me and told me that he understood what I was going through which made me lose control all over again. How could he possibly know what I was going through? If he knew what I was going through, why would he have destroyed the evidence? He proceeded to explain that as the diary was of no monetary value, they'd made the decision to destroy it. Monetary value? Does blood or semen evidence have any monetary value? Just because it wasn't millions of dollars in cash, didn't mean it didn't have value.

I asked him if he'd actually read it. He refused to give me a distinct answer. I asked him if the diary had been scanned and copies kept on file in case the rapist struck again. I told the officer the rapist had already tried to rape another person. Again, he refused to give me an answer.

My husband fortunately had the forethought to tell the officer he wanted an email stating his version of what had happened. We left the office, and I was completely obliterated. I don't even remember heading back to the office to get our things and walk home. I know I stayed in my bed for days, sobbing every time I woke up. We did receive the email from the officer with a very basic apology and stating why he'd decided to destroy the evidence.

I desperately wanted to know if there were any copies on file of the diary, something no one would answer, so I contacted a friend of a relative who was a police officer and explained what had happened. He was horrified and agreed that evidence into anything of a sexual nature of a minor is not supposed to ever be destroyed. As I had the case number details, he was able to look at the case on the police system and told me there was a PDF file attached to the case, but he could not open it as it would be risking his job. I absolutely did not want to do that.

My complaint went all the way to the Police Ombudsman twice. I was told to file a Freedom of Information application to find out if the PDF file was a copy of the diary, but it was denied as they said it was not mine.

I was devastated and thoroughly exhausted and decided that I had to let the fight go. I couldn't afford a lawyer. I had absolutely no proof I could access and none of it was going to bring my daughter back. I made the decision to put my efforts into helping other parents who were struggling with their teens, and to do more research so I could talk to people, politicians, journalists – absolutely anyone who would listen.

The whole experience completely rocked my world. My faith in humanity was at an all time low. I couldn't trust people, I couldn't trust the government, I certainly couldn't trust so-called medical professionals and I could no longer trust the police. It's a very strange feeling to be in that space. I felt so alone, so apart from the rest of society, but it was also strangely liberating. I'd been hurt so badly by everyone around me, how much worse could it get? I no longer felt like the good law abiding citizen who blindly did as I was told, and I questioned absolutely everything, every bit of information, every suggested health advice. Trust the science? I don't think so!

Christmas came and went. It felt like there was very little to celebrate. I didn't know where my daughter was, if she was safe and healthy. I pushed myself to try and get into the spirit for the sake of my son.

I decided I couldn't face being at home for my daughter's 18th birthday and not be able to see her. It was such a milestone to miss out on. We decided to go on a holiday, far away from our home so that I was in a different environment. The day before her birthday, I received a phone call from my daughter. I couldn't believe it. I answered the phone cautiously. I didn't know what to say.

The conversation was a little strained, with me trying not to cry. I asked her where she was and asked her whether she was safe etc. She said she'd been staying at a trans friend's house initially, but they'd dropped her off at a youth homeless shelter because they hadn't been getting on. I was furious! The activist who'd tried to take her from our home, finally succeeded in getting her out, only to dump her in a homeless shelter?

She asked me what I was doing the next day (her birthday). I decided to stick to the complete truth and I told her that as she hadn't contacted me at all and that she was with her new friends, I'd assumed that she wouldn't want to see me on her birthday and being that I couldn't cope with not seeing her, we'd gone away. She told me none of her new friends had been in contact with her for weeks. No one was going to be there for her birthday. This aspect really infuriates me. The activists steal these vulnerable traumatised youth from their families, and then when it gets too hard, they dump them! No wonder the suicide rate goes up!

Fortunately, I was able to tell my daughter that her Grandma would love to see her and to call her and then when I returned home, we could celebrate too. I felt like the world's worst mother, but at least she wasn't going to be alone.

I was able to see her the following month. She was exactly as she'd been when she left home at this point, but with shorter hair. My husband did not want to see her, so my mother, my son and I met her at a café for her birthday. My son was excited to see his sister as they'd always been very close. Things were going very well until my daughter went into the men's bathroom with my son and he freaked out. No way was he going into the bathroom with his sister and how could she just walk into the men's bathroom? We parted ways with her promising to keep in touch.

I would send my daughter photos and anything of interest via text messages to keep in touch with her as she wasn't really keeping in touch with me. I felt that at least if I could see she was reading the messages, I knew she was alive and basically OK.

I received a call from her again a couple of months later that rocked me. Her name had come up on my phone and worried and excited to talk to her, I answered only to have someone with a completely different voice answer me. I knew she'd planned to start taking testosterone after the age of 18, but I hadn't realised just how quickly the change of voice would take place. I didn't believe it was her initially. I literally thought someone was playing tricks or had found her phone. Can you imagine not recognising your own child's voice, or realising that the changes are permanent, so that you'd never hear that voice again? It was a huge hurdle for me to cope with.

I was also of course devastated that she had started taking the hormones for the other myriad of health issues, and the fact that I could not imagine my beautiful daughter with a receding hairline and facial hair.

One day, I decided to log into my daughter's old computer that she'd left here on the off chance that I could find some sort of information there about the rape and the grooming by the teacher. Although there was no evidence as such, what I did find was that she had created multiple email accounts which had been used to open up various social media accounts that I knew nothing about.

Her internet browser history showed that she'd been on a website called Depression Quest regularly. I'd never heard of it before and I thought it might have been something to help her deal with her depression, but it was the opposite.

Depression Quest is described as a Freeware game started in 2013 and is described as a "interactive Fiction Game". It actually comes with a warning that it may cause depression! It gives scenarios where you can make a variety of choices for how you'd deal with a situation, giving positive and negative answers, or could they be clues to teach youth about how to act more depressed?

I started talking to other parents about their teen's usage of this game, and it appears to be something that is common within the ROGD cohort of teens. Could this be why when my daughter started telling the police she was in 'emotional danger' and suicidal that she was using language that wasn't her own?

There was also a great deal of time being spent on a site called Deviart. When my daughter had asked me about 18 months beforehand if she could start an account, I had looked at it, and thought it looked ok. It featured various people's artwork, much of which were anime characters, and videos giving lessons on how to draw. My daughter had studied Japanese at school and was quite into Anime and she loved to draw. There had been a rash of parents who'd mentioned Deviart so I decided to set up an account. Once I'd gotten in, I made my way to a chat area, thinking it would be discussions about art. It was definitely not art related, it was clear grooming and very disturbing. There were members complaining about non affirming parents, and other older sounding members telling them that what their parents were doing (by non-affirming, deadnaming, misgendering) was abuse and that they should leave as soon as possible.

There was a whole chat feed devoted to giving the angry activist type answers to comments on social media. How to convince Christian parents that the bible is wrong saying there's only two genders, and a (very weird) thread about the concept of cracking an egg. This theory says that every person who is not transgender is an uncracked egg. Inside them is the 'queerness' just waiting to come out, and you just have to crack the egg hard enough for the person to realise. So in other words, everyone is transgender, we just don't know about it yet.

There was another thread where peers were teaching newly hatched transgender teens that the way to get what they wanted from their parents and medical professionals was to act depressed. It mentioned Depression Quest as a way to learn to act genuinely depressed. It went into so much detail about things like not going onto a particular type of antidepressant, because it could get rid of gender dysphoria! It detailed the types of side effects and symptoms to mention to the doctor so they would swap to another antidepressant.

It was here I also learned about Furries (anthropomorphic animals, or animals with human qualities) and went down some very deep dark holes of graphic pornography drawings with animals with human features. Different furry personas have different kinks from paedophilia to 'pee play', to bondage. It was sickening and shocking to say the least.

My horrible research did go to good use with helping some people going through court cases.

I learned that learning Japanese at schools can be detrimental to children as it can introduce them to this world of anime where many of the characters are highly sexualised, transgender, and furries. School pornography filters are not able to filter out the pornographic anime content from the innocent content, so children can literally watch this anime porn while at school. Furries, like transgender, have strong communities which are very sexualised and disturbing. (It's interesting that over the time of researching all this matter, teens are now identifying as cats and dogs even in Australian schools).

For the next few months, I only really heard from my daughter when she needed something. As she'd turned 18, she was asked to leave the youth homeless shelter and she moved into another type of accommodation for youths up to the age of 25. She called me and asked me to help her move. The flat she was given was clean and neat and furnished and seemed very safe, but she lacked all the different items needed to set up a house – sheets, towels, kitchen items etc. Of course I took her out and bought her all the items she needed. The accommodation came with rules, one was that you had to be in full time education, working or looking for work. As my daughter refused to do any of those things, she was eventually kicked out.

Her next move was to a share house with other young adults, this time with no sort of supervision or rules. Her room here was not furnished so I bought her what she needed. I was also concerned that she would not have the backup support at this 'normal' share house compared to her last more structured accommodation. At the same time, I wondered whether a less supportive environment might be better for her, because there would be less contact with those people pushing the trans agenda. As per her previous accommodation, once she was settled and had everything she needed, she stopped communicating again.

A couple of months later I received another call for help as she'd been kicked out of her accommodation again. She would not tell me the reason for her being kicked out but she left most of her belongings again claiming she couldn't find them. She said her bed had been broken and the wardrobe I had purchased was gone.

The next accommodation was with a male who had a job and I hoped for a better outcome for her. The fact that her flatmate was older and employed sounded promising and scary at the same time for me. Communication was again sporadic.

After months of absolutely no communication again, I decided to go to her home and make sure she was ok. The male that answered the door looked really uncomfortable when I told him who I was. I managed to find out that she'd been in hospital but was now out and staying with friends. I was very worried about her obviously, with the added layer of being terrified that she'd had her breasts removed. When I asked if he knew if she was at a particular friend's house, he said yes. Worried and not sure what to do, my mother and I decided to go to the friend's place who turned out to be the original boy who was transitioning to female that she'd started dating. My experience of his mother was that she was an interfering, manipulative and toxic woman.

I was extremely concerned about going to this house. I was worried about my reaction to seeing this awful person. My anxiety levels were through the roof. This mum had caused us so much harm. There were no cars in the driveway so we decided to park and knock on the door. We could hear noises inside and the house was not locked up so we kept knocking and waiting, trying to get a glimpse of our girl.

A few moments later, the boy my daughter was dating walked down the driveway and asked what we wanted. We told him we were not going until we'd spoken to my daughter. He went into the house and came back a few minutes later saying that 'he' didn't want to see anyone. My mum simply said tough and pushed through the door with me close behind her calling my daughter's name. We found my daughter in bed, looking very bashful about being caught out.

I was so relieved, I burst into tears and hugged her. We held each other for ages and I asked her if she was ok and what had been happening. She explained that she hadn't been in a good place and had just got out of hospital. Other than looking bashful, my daughter looked fine. She was giggling and not appearing at all depressed. I begged her to promise me she'd keep in touch and we left.

For a couple of weeks she kept her promise. She told me one day that she was going into a mental health facility again and told me not to worry if she didn't respond to my messages. She asked that we bring snacks if we came to visit which we did the following day. It was a high security facility where we had to leave our bags, take off bangles and watches and take off any shoes with laces. We were told we could see her in an interview room where we would be observed. I was apprehensive, but at the same time relieved that they were taking her mental health so seriously.

When my daughter came into the room, she was again, perfectly normal. Chatting about the normal everyday things we talked about. I could see no signs of depression. She laughed, made jokes etc. I was happy to hear that they were only allowed their mobile phones for an hour in the evenings, so if I messaged her, she would respond then. I was very excited about this. Taking her away from the outside influences on social media was something I'd been trying to do. I felt it was very positive. With promises to see her again soon, we left.

The next day, my phone rang and I was surprised to see it was my daughter calling at a time when she wasn't supposed to be on her phone. She sounded as if she was outside. After she'd asked me a couple of questions, I decided to ask her why she was allowed to call me from her phone at this time. What she told me completely blew me away! She said she'd needed to buy some things from the shop, so they'd allowed her to go out UNATTENDED, WITHOUT SUPERVISION. So the night before, my Mum and I had been told to take off bangles and shoes with laces because my daughter was so suicidal, but here she was completely alone and out in the general public with access to absolutely anything. How can they be so concerned about her one night, and allow her out the very next morning? I couldn't understand. She was discharged a couple of days later.

We kept in contact for a while at this point and my daughter told me she'd been accepted into a mental health residential program where troubled teens went to learn how to take care of themselves, cook, do washing and get into a routine. She would be there for one month and had her own small unit within the complex.

I was so frustrated. My daughter was not a child raised by a drug addict who hadn't taught her all of life's basics. She knew how to cook, she knew how to look after herself, she just wasn't motivated to do so. How was this going to help her with her rape trauma? Although it might be a really helpful program for some teens, I didn't know how it would benefit her, but at least she was safe and moving in a positive direction. She called and messaged frequently during this time and we visited her a couple of times a week, taking her out for lunch and just connecting with her.

During this time, she broke up with the boy who'd been transitioning. I was really pleased. Breaking up with him meant less interference with the boy's mum, and hopefully would give her a chance to meet some new people who would be a positive influence in her life.

More and more I was starting to see my 'old daughter', not the gender influenced activist she'd become. You see, as part of being 'male' my daughter had been doing all the stereotypical male actions for her male persona. Burping loudly, passing wind loudly, eating enormous amounts of food like her younger brother was prone to do, except that she would eat until she actually vomited and then half an hour later, wanted more food. She had never acted in this way before transitioning. It was embarrassing to be with her in public sometimes when she was doing her male 'performance'. The change in her personality with her transitioning had been profound. One day, while shopping, my daughter wanted to try on a dress. She ended up buying it. She told me she was still male, but a feminine male. Ok, I didn't care, it was one step closer to being her old self.

I was pushing myself to use her new chosen name because it was gender neutral. It was so hard to do, but I thought it was worth it to have her in my life. I avoided pronoun use all together.

Right at the end of her residential stay, she told me she'd got back together with her old trans woman boyfriend. I tried to remain hopeful that the previous couple of weeks where we'd really reconnected would be enough to remind her that I loved her and to stay in touch so we could have a relationship.

Again, I believe thanks to the transwoman boyfriend and his mum's influence, communication faded right out again. The messages went from being 'my daughter' to this trans activist persona again. She would criticise anything and everything I said or not respond at all. When she did respond, I strongly believe the messages were written by someone else. The vocabulary and sentence structure was completely different.

One day out of the blue, she contacted my mother and asked if she could stay with her for a couple of weeks as she had nowhere else to go. The boyfriend's mum had decided she didn't want her there any more. My Mum lives in a tiny unit, so it would be awkward, but she took her in.

It was a very difficult time for my Mum with my daughter being up all night and keeping her awake. She would prepare snacks during the night and leave her mess everywhere. She refused to help with anything or help to pay for food. My Mum just kept trying to help her find a place and be kind to her. She ended up staying for about 2 months and then moved out to another unknown location.

My daughter decided to come to our home for Christmas that year. By this stage, we'd had a couple of Christmases without her and I'd been miserable. Along with the trans persona, my daughter had become a militant vegan and so I prepared her a comprehensive vegan meal I thought she would appreciate. I bought her useful gifts that were non gender specific, things I hoped she would find useful. What I hadn't contemplated was my husband and son's reaction to her being in our home again. It was not happy families.

My husband could barely bring himself to look at her, and my son refused to even be in the same room. I was angry with my husband, how could he not be excited that she was in our home again? I was devastated for my son though. He was a young teen and was so angry and upset that he literally paced the house like some animal at the zoo. He was so furious he could barely talk. How dare she be in this house he kept asking me - she's not part of this family any more. He wouldn't even open presents! I begged him just to keep his cool until she was gone, which he was able to do (sort of). The tension was so thick you could have cut through it with a knife. We had an early lunch because my daughter had planned to visit her trans woman boyfriend. She proceeded to eat everything on the table, largely ignoring her carefully produced vegan food. I honestly wonder now if she did it to make it as awkward as possible for me. After my daughter left, my son collapsed into bed and slept for hours. I decided I couldn't put my son through that again and vowed that I would see my daughter when he was not at home or out of the house.

My son and I talked later. I had been in such a world of pain that I didn't really consider what my poor son had been going through. He and my husband were furious that my daughter had hurt me so much and then had the gall to come into the house without any sort of apology or anything else and expect everyone to just keep going as if nothing had happened. You see, my son and husband had witnessed my breakdowns, the agony of going on without my daughter, the worry and the stress she caused me. They both had taken a bit of a back seat where my life had become a shell where I'd stopped doing anything I enjoyed and was glued to the phone and computer, talking to other parents and trying to figure out a way to save our children. My son was grieving that the sister he'd loved had completely dumped him. Again, that was my fault. In the early days, my daughter had told me she was going to explain the transgender movement to my son and I'd stopped her. I had told her literally over my dead body was she going to try and influence him and convert him to think that transitioning was ok.

In my son's school life, he was getting grief about his thoughts on the transgender movement, and it was influencing his friendships and relationships. He was called a bigot and transphobic etc too because he didn't tolerate people who pushed the transgender agenda. He'd learned his sister had been raped and by whom and so he did not want to sit in a class and be taught the highly sexualised content of many of his health lessons. He didn't want to talk about acceptance and diversity. He'd personally experienced the pain of his sister being so hurt and manipulated.

There were some students in his school who were non-binary and the school had allowed them to wear sports uniforms instead of the more constrictive formal uniforms the other students had to wear. One morning he got ready for school wearing his sports uniform. When I questioned what he was doing, he'd responded that if the non-binary kids could do it, so would he. I couldn't talk him out of it, so I decided it was his form of activism so I let him go. I was sent emails from the school telling me that he'd been in the incorrect uniform for no good reason so he would receive a detention. The next morning, sports uniform again. More emails and then in the coming days, phone calls from school telling me I had to stop him. I refused. One morning the school counsellor called me. She wanted to find out what was going on.

I told the counsellor at length about what had happened to his sister and how I thought this was my son's coping mechanism, a protest to show the non-binary kids were getting special privileges, and to get back at the students who thought he was transphobic.

To my utmost horror, the counsellor after listening to our story actually said she didn't understand what the issue was because there was nothing wrong with some children transitioning. 'Better a live son than a dead daughter' again. I saw red! I stopped the conversation and told her that I would no longer take calls from her and that I would withdraw any sort of implied consent that she had to talk to my son alone from that time on as I was horrified that she accepted what I felt was tantamount to child abuse. I did email the school formally after the conversation and explained my thoughts and actions.

My son calmly accepted his daily detentions saying he didn't care, at least he was in air conditioned comfort, and kept up his protest for about 3 weeks. While I was so worried about him at the time, I was also so proud of his strength of conviction.

I had expected to be able to see my daughter for her birthday as she'd been ok with me at Christmas, but she didn't want to see me, but agreed to meet at a shopping centre when I told her I had a present for her.

From that point on, all my messages were ignored. There was no sign that she'd even read them. Covid started and along with that, the great supermarket shortages and unprecedented toilet paper shortages. I was concerned for my daughter. She had managed to get onto a disability pension so didn't have a great deal of ready cash. She didn't drive and I didn't know if she had access to a car to be able to go to different supermarkets to get the things she needed. As I'd always bought in bulk, I messaged her asking her how she was and if she needed anything. No response. I tried again a week later saying I had enough toilet paper to share and some of the staple foods she used. I told her she didn't have to visit with me, I could just drop it off to her and leave or leave it at someone's house if she'd rather. No response. This was repeated every couple of weeks for a few months until I was so sick with worry for her I messaged her and poured my heart out, saying that I didn't know what I'd done wrong, and if she didn't want to have contact with me, that was fine, but I was just worried about her welfare and could she just let me know she was ok. No response again. I didn't know what to do.

Suddenly a couple of weeks later, I received notification of a message from her. I was super excited to hear from her! The message however was devastating. She told me that I was a horribly abusive parent and that I was emotionally blackmailing her. She told me that I was so toxic that I made her sick and she didn't want to hear from me again. There was so much hate and loathing in that message, it took my breath away. I still don't know what I did wrong. Sharing what I had with other people was not a new thing for me, so it wasn't as if it should have surprised her that I'd offered to share what we had. I did respond and told her that I didn't understand what I'd done to deserve such hatred from her, but I told her that I still loved her and that I would still always be here if she needed me.

Life goes on so they say, and so did ours, but without my daughter. I was constantly worried about her. I went through many nightmares of looking for her in a crowd of people with no faces. Covid lockdowns and issues meant that I homeschooled my son and I ran myself completely ragged.

My parent support group was growing as more distressed parents reached out to try and get some assistance. Some weeks I would receive up to 14 new parent introductions. I would get phone calls from distressed parents who'd just found out their children were having breasts or a penis removed. How could they stop their children from harming themselves? How could doctors and mental health professionals not investigate thoroughly about the issues that had been occurring in these teen's lives and see that they needed true mental health, not amputation of healthy body tissue? They all hoped I had a miracle cure, a magic wand; of course there were none. Some days I felt like giving it all up. What worth was I bringing to these parents? I couldn't save my daughter, so what did I have to offer them? Then I would receive a message from a parent thanking me for what I was doing and I'd pull myself up and keep going.

I was barely working in a paid capacity at this time. There were always urgent matters, parents in distress, people who needed guidance and assistance. My activism work became everything to me and it helped me to deal with my pain. I felt that if I could at least help someone else save their child, or help lawyers to win cases that would change the laws, my grief and unique set of knowledge would have been worth it. Our family suffered because of it, including financially. It's hard to spend 40 hours a week doing activism and helping parents etc and then still fit in a paid job as well as running a household and being a wife and mother. It was exhausting, but it somehow almost kept me going. It impacted greatly on our social life too. How could I go to a party or function or have people over when I was so triggered by the loss of my daughter? I was doing so much deep, dark investigation that I felt that I had nothing to talk about in these situations. I'd stopped all my hobbies, I had zero interest in work, the only thing that mattered was this, and it's not exactly party or dinner table conversation. We stopped entertaining at home. I was too exhausted, too broken and too broke to be able to have dinner parties which I used to love to do. I lost my confidence completely.

It was hard looking at posts on social media from my daughter's old friend's parents. School balls, graduation, drivers licence, jobs. I missed all those milestones.

During this time, I've had a great deal of growth in many areas, and faced many fears and challenges. One of the hardest things I had to do was speak to a transgender person. After my experience with the trans activists, I was hesitant (to say the least) to have to speak to one.

I was asked by someone I was helping if I knew any trans people who might be against the transitioning of children. Yes I did! I'd been following Scott Newgent online for some time.

I messaged Scott and shortly after he responded via a video call. I was terrified, but determined, so I answered the call. Scott was surprisingly easy to talk to. He is against children transitioning and was sympathetic when I told him what we'd gone through with our daughter. He was happy to help and put me in contact with a more local transgender person. Again, overcoming my fears I reached out and met Kevin, who I ended up speaking to for hours! I was truly amazed that we had so much to talk about, so much in common. As I got to know Kevin better, I was able to listen to issues from his unique point of view which was fascinating to say the least. Better still was that I was able to ask him all the nitty gritty questions a parent of a child who is transitioning wants to know. Kevin has been a Godsend, not only for me, but in speaking with other parents who also had lots of weird and wonderful questions. You see, Kevin is quite different from transgender teens like my daughter and her friends, and also the teens of other parents I'd spoken to. Kevin isn't an activist and he's not coming after anyone's children. He's also very happy to listen to concerns.

As time went on, I became more and more worried about my daughter and not hearing from her. I had no clue where she was. One day out of the blue she sent me an SMS with just a link to a website she'd created before blocking me again so I couldn't respond.

The website showed clearly that my poor daughter was not doing well. The website was basically just about her and the rules of how to deal and communicate with her. She listed a set of disabilities she supposedly had – weird and wonderful things I'd never heard of before. These disabilities supposedly explained why she couldn't keep her space tidy (she couldn't bend over), that she was a witch and that she was also part alien. Let's forget the witch and alien part for a moment..... My daughter had been doing dance since she was 3. She was very active and talented. If she'd had any sort of physical disability it would have been picked up a long time ago!

It was clear from one of the photos she sent me when she first ran away that she had gotten into the occult, as the photo showed her wearing a pentagram, with a shaved head, and wearing heavy black eye-shadow. It made me extremely worried about her. As was the fact that she was describing herself as an alien on her website.

About this time, a friend who also had a child wanting to transition, bumped into my daughter's Go Fund Me page. My daughter had created it early on in the hopes of getting enough money together to have her breasts amputated. The page had been updated to say that my daughter had raised enough money for the surgery and was going to see a local surgeon whose name she mentioned. I was horrified but as I had the surgeon's name, I decided to write to him and let him know about her history of mental instability and trauma and try to get him not to do the surgery.

I contacted a therapist I had become friends with over the previous few years and asked him to look at the website she'd created and see if he thought it was as bad as I did. My worst fears were confirmed; he was of the firm view that she would be unable to consent to surgery in what was obviously a very troubled mental state.

I wrote to the surgeon, giving him screenshots of her website, her background story and history and the fact that she'd never had trauma counselling to help her get over the rape trauma. The office manager who responded to my emails was very sympathetic and I was hopeful that it would be enough to stop the surgery.

The doctor eventually wrote me to say that he thought she was fine, but would send her for a session with a psychiatrist to make sure. He'd listed the name of this psychiatrist and it was one that worked in the gender clinic, so of course he wouldn't find a reason to stop her having the surgery.

I received a very angry text message again from my daughter, with so much toxic abuse I couldn't believe it. She stated that the doctor had given her my emails (he had kindly printed them out for her), and that she was effectively disowning me. I was furious at the doctor interfering in such a way! I reported him to AHPRA (Australian Health Practitioner Regulation Agency), which was another long and painful process. Of course, in my opinion, AHPRA has been completely captured by the trans agenda and so after a long process of report writing, they ended up saying he'd done nothing wrong.

My daughter had stated the date of the surgery and it was coming up in a matter of weeks. I decided to do a letter campaign to all the hospitals in our city where she might go for this surgery. Many people joined in and together we sent a couple of hundred letters to the hospitals, enough that I received calls from a couple of the heads of hospital stating they had no control about whether a person should be able to consent or not.

The surgery day loomed like a ticking time bomb. I felt as if it was an execution. My beautiful, perfect daughter was amputating body parts. I was also furious that at the time, all non essential surgery had been cancelled and yet the surgeon who was going to take my daughter's breasts was still doing lists of girls having their breast amputated in the name of the trans movement and to supposedly improve their mental health.

I didn't think I would be able to survive it. I actually went to the doctor and asked for help. I wanted something that would just knock me out so I didn't know what was happening. It felt like the end of the world. Some of you reading this may think I'm overreacting, but I know that it's something all the parents going through this feel. It's like a full stop. The end of the fight, the end of our child as we know it. It may not be rational, but to us it's the end. Mercifully, I survived it. On the day, I slept mostly and woke up sobbing, remembering why I felt as if there was a hole in my chest.

Just to rub salt in the wound, the day after surgery, my daughter sent a photo to my poor mother of her with her mutilated chest and fresh cutting marks all over her arms. My daughter told my mother that she was furious with me, because the head of the hospital she'd attended came and spoke to her during her admission about the number of letters that had been written to try and stop the surgery. I was quietly pleased in one way….at least she knew I was thinking of her. The message to my mother seemed to snap me out of my funk somehow. Yes, she no longer had breasts, but nothing else, especially not her attitude had changed.

As my reputation grew within the community, so did the parents seeking help with other issues too, issues of gross government overreach, of schools grooming and keeping secrets about their children. School councillors who played God and would call Child Protection Services when a mother was punishing her own teen by confiscating their phone! Phones apparently have become a human right and a mother should not remove a phone under any circumstances. One mother bought a new basic phone to replace her child's phone, only to have a call from Child Services the next day saying they would start a case unless she gave her child the original smart phone. How has a mobile phone owned by a parent, paid for by the parents, suddenly become a human right?

Some parents found out their child was 'trans' by accident when attending graduation ceremonies and seeing their child's photo on the screen with a different opposite sex name. Some received school reports with the wrong name on it. How can children appear happy in their natal sex in their home and extracurricular life but be the opposite sex at school?

I was asked to speak at different events and made sure I organised in-person meetings with the parents in my support group along the way. Many of these parents have become like my soul sisters. We've exposed our truths, our pain in the most brutally honest way to a virtual stranger and we've connected because of it. People can think what they like, but until they have personally experienced the pain, the confusion, the grief of the whole foundation of your world changing, they just can't understand. It's why parent support groups are so important to parents. I've given my phone number to every parent in my group, and I've had many emergency calls. Calls about 'glitter parents' trying to take their child, calls about blow ups that have happened between family members, marriages that have broken up because of differences on how to handle their child, or just the inability to get through the grief of losing a child to this movement; calls about police taking children, calls that their child is having surgery as they speak and they need someone to pour out their pain to. Calls that they feel like they just can't keep going on in this crazy, upside down, dystopian world. I have spoken to probably thousands of (mainly) mums, from literally around the world. Hong Kong, New Zealand, Italy, Germany, Sweden, UK, US, Canada, Israel and Singapore. It amazes me still that we are all experiencing the same craziness and that our children are following the same steps to get what they want.

My dream from early on was to start an organisation where we could help parents and detransitioners in a more formal way. As I'd witnessed parents going through court cases to try and save their children from detransitioning I'd seen not only the emotional and mental cost to these families, but the financial costs too. Although a few lawyers were taking these cases pro bono, the court process is still hugely expensive. I'd tried desperately to help these families drum up financial support for these families and the lawyers too, but while public funding platforms such as GoFundMe are happy to fundraise for teens to have surgeries to cut off healthy body tissue, they're not willing to help parents fight for custody of their children. I approached a number of large well known free speech type organisations to help with funding, but they were all unwilling to stick their necks out into the fray of the transgender movement. While supporting sportsmen (for example) was appealing to many because it was so black and white and reportable, supporting parents who are completely gagged by the courts with these awful situations doesn't bring enough reportable publicity. While I did have some overseas organisations willing to send some money for these cases, without an organisation the money transfer process and subsequent tax implications made it impossible. I hoped that starting an organisation which actually provided on-the-ground, practical help for parents would attract supporters.

I was very fortunate to be introduced to a powerhouse woman who had the same idea as I did towards the end of 2022. This friend has all sorts of amazing skills and experience that I just didn't have to be able to make this dream a reality. We were able to combine our unique knowledgebase, skill set and work ethic to start to do some actual practical, concrete work to support parents. It is very early days, but we have already had some significant moments.

I've spent hours and hours of my life contacting media, politicians, parenting 'experts', activists, feminists, lawyers, researchers, anyone who might be able to help get the word out that our children are being harmed. Most emails go unanswered, most phone messages ignored, or worse, someone says they want to talk to you. They interview you for hours, bringing up the pain over and over and then at the end say that they're sorry, but it's just too complex to take anywhere.

What we've been asking and begging for is an independent review of the gender industry in Australia. We don't want a review chaired by activists, or gender affirming doctors, but one with a sensible group of unbiased, scientific professionals to thoroughly review what's happening in Australia. In the UK, they had what is now known as The Cass Review which brought to light the medical malpractice in the Tavistock Centre there. We are confident that if an unbiased professional was to really review what's happening in Australia, it would be clear that there is no scientific basis in how they are dealing with patients with gender dysphoria.

I'm happy to report that since working on this writing, there has been a huge event unfold. The World Professional Association for Transgender Health (WPATH) who are the world recognised leaders in developing guidelines for gender affirming care have had a series of documents and videos leaked to the public. In Australia, and in most countries around the world, these WPATH guidelines have been used extensively as a basis for each country's standards of care. In Australia The Australian Professional Association for Trans Health (AUSPATH), described as "the peak body of professionals involved in the health, rights and well-being of all trans people, binary and non-binary", uses the WPATH Guidelines extensively for their own set of guidelines.

What these documents and files show is very questionable ethical practices suggesting that WPATH members may have proceeded with treatment protocols despite potential long term adverse side effects, especially with children and vulnerable adults. There are questions regarding 'informed consent' (Defined in the Oxford Dictionary as "permission granted in full knowledge of the possible consequences, typically that which is given by a patient to a doctor for treatment with knowledge of the possible risks and benefits"). Concerns are raised that patients' understanding of the long term consequences of gender affirming treatments is inadequate. The files also point to a lack of consideration for the long term outcomes for patients undergoing treatment, with some practices described as experimental and without scientific backing. Some of the documents that have been leaked show cancer developing in the livers of very young patients, something that shouldn't take a scientist to work out should not be happening. Hormone Replacement Therapy used to be commonplace amongst menopausal women, until the link between these treatments and cancers came to light. Nowadays, it's very difficult for women to access synthetic drugs for menopause symptoms and if they are given, it's for very short periods of time. Transgender patients are given much higher doses of synthetic wrong sex hormones and we are finding they are often given with medication such as Spirolactone which helps to reduce levels of testosterone. One mother discovered her young adult son on 4 times the recommended amount of this drug as well as wrong sex hormones prescribed to transition her son. Looking up this drug, there have been studies shown stating significant side effects from its use, especially from such large doses.

From a parent whose daughter has been on testosterone for years and already had her breasts amputated, the news was bittersweet. While most are ecstatic that what they've been trying to scream from the rooftops regarding the damage has been confirmed, any changes made at this point are obviously too late for my daughter, and many other parent's children. Reading through the files the night they were released I was devastated, and furious. These people, these 'experts' knew they were harming children, yet the 'medical professionals' in the gender clinics and other clinics mocked us for questioning the safety of their guidelines. They mocked us for stating basic biology. No one is ever born in the wrong body, and no human has ever changed sex. As a transexual friend of mine says, of course I'm still a woman. I just look very different than most. It's been almost 4 years since I spoke to my daughter. I miss her every day. I miss the person she was and the relationship we had. I mourn for the loss of the relationship with her sibling, I mourn for the experiences she has missed and will never get back and I worry constantly for her health and mental wellbeing. I ache to hug her. I ache to listen to her laugh. Parenting was never meant to be this difficult or this crazy. What I do know is that I'll never stop fighting to protect all the people being harmed by this dreadful agenda. What the professionals, activists, and the children themselves forget is to never get between a mother and her young (regardless of age, our protective instincts will always be there), and that when hopefully these lost youth realise they've made a massive mistake, it won't be the medical professionals or the activists or their glitter families that will be there to help them. It will be the mums and dads waiting to help them heal.

CHAPTER 3

Tara's story

When my eldest daughter, Grace, told me in tears that she was trans, I was confused.

When she later told me in a hollow robotic voice with glassy eyes that she needed to have top surgery and start taking testosterone to live an authentic life, I was terrified.

Terrified of failing in my most sacred duty as a mother. To protect my children from harm.

My fears are well founded. And our family's situation is far from unique.

Both my daughters have fallen victim to the modern mania of transgenderism.

The last three years have been a plodding kind of hell lit by spotlights of hope.

Not long after Grace told me she thought she was trans, my younger daughter, Claire, told me she was convinced she was trapped in the wrong body. And only a gender transition could set her free.

Tens of thousands of young women just like Grace and Claire are identifying as trans, usually as part of an online or school-based friendship group.

They are at great risk of harm. Harm disguised as help.

But how did this happen? And what can we do?

Well, through careful listening, open-minded research and trusting my gut, I've worked some of it out.

On 26 January 2020 – Australia Day – my family (myself, my husband, and our two daughters) attended a barbeque at the beach. We were celebrating our baby nephew's first birthday. It is a lovely memory. A time from a lost world. A world before Grace changed. A time before Covid.

We enjoyed the day very much, eating sausages, drinking wine, chatting with relatives and laughing as the baby continued the family tradition of putting his fist into his birthday cake and then consuming it with gusto after smearing it around as widely as possible.

My dear first-born daughter, Grace, was sixteen, and she was so beautiful. She wore her brand-new gingham one piece swimsuit. Her long blonde hair slid over her milky white shoulders as she relaxed in the sun. I fretted on her perfect pale skin burning and on the admiring glances she was receiving from young passing men. She stretched and yawned like a cat, enjoying the extent of her slender young frame. Her body. Grace had become a woman.

How I envied her. I was once that lovely too.

I felt the first pangs of loss then. Realising that Grace was growing up and would soon want to leave home.

Oh, I had no idea of the storm that was brewing!

A dangerous new virus had been detected in Wuhan. Little did we realise at that lovely sunshiney family barbeque that our lives were about to change irreparably.

Then in March 2020, my father died.

The dangerous new virus now had a name, Covid, and it was definitely more serious than the Avian Flu and the Swine Flu that had preceded it.

My father had always been a practical joker and dropping dead in Scotland in the early days of a global pandemic was a masterstroke. Sometimes I think he was just leaving early to avoid the traffic.

I flew to Scotland for Dad's funeral, dismissing the escalating chorus of concern over Covid as alarmist. In the background of my father's funeral and a thoroughly Scottish wake, the anxious calls to return home grew louder.

I am still astonished at how blasé I was. Surely Australia wouldn't actually shut its borders? Who knew that the borders would remain shut for twenty long months as the virus burned a deadly path around the world?

As the science fiction fan that I am, I sometimes dwell on the thought that there is an alternate universe where I stayed shut out of Australia and my poor husband had to handle Grace's gathering mental health crisis on his own.

Australia fared better than most other countries in the pandemic. I feel that we carry survivor guilt over this. And, like the after-effects and side-effects of Covid, it manifests itself in many ways.

In the Australian public health arsenal, the greatest weapon against Covid was lockdowns. If you could stay at home, you had to stay at home. The constrictions on personal freedom of movement squeezed tighter and tighter. We itched and chafed and grumbled but, for the most part, complied.

And it worked. Our Covid numbers were contained. Our death rate stayed low.

Of course, everyone's lockdown experience was different. Some bore it with good grace, being temperamentally well-suited to the isolation. But some paced in their cages like panthers at the zoo.

And our kids suddenly had too much time and too much internet on their hands.

During the lockdowns, Grace started self-diagnosing her anxieties on the internet. She used them as labels in her social media profile. These diagnoses, real or imaginary, soothed her anxieties with certainties. They gave her excuses for her more difficult behaviours. They gave her a point of commonality with others and helped her to form her own online tribe.

They also planted flags that would attract 'Pam'.

Grace met 'Pam' on a Discord server. Grace poured out her heart about how bad her life was, how uncertain she felt in her own body, and how bleak the future seemed.

'Pam' responded with, "that's how I felt before I realised I was trans."

And my poor daughter fell down a digital rabbit hole.

In April 2020, Grace declared that she knew what was 'wrong' with her. She announced that she was a man and intended to transition her gender.

Scared and confused though we were, my husband and I did our best to keep our heads and to be supportive. In the privacy of our bedroom, we held each other and whispered our confused theories. What was happening to Grace? A lovely young girl who had been luxuriating in the sun in a gingham one-piece bathing suit only a few months earlier.

Grace shaved off her long blond hair and adopted a skater-boi style. She tore everything out of her room and threw away almost all records of herself as a child. She sought to lay a fresh path in the future by destroying evidence of her past. She declared her birth name to be a 'dead name'. She threw out all her clothes and replaced them with men's clothes. She adopted a deep voice and would swagger about. She would man-spread when she sat down.

Even in the early days of the pandemic, the strain on mental health services was acute and growing. I talked to our doctor, and she referred Grace to a psychologist under a Mental Health Care Plan. Grace was initially willing to engage with the only psychologist we could access.

The psychologist confessed to me that she was stumped. Grace was ticking a lot of boxes across a lot of checklists but could not be definitively diagnosed with any known mental disorder. The psychologist recommended that Grace see a psychiatrist.

Things got worse and worse. Grace dropped out of high school. Always a smart, but lazy kid content to skive along on her good memory, she never studied much but did okay. Suddenly it was all too much.

Her temper worsened. She made false accusations of abuse against us to her psychologist. She would shout at me that I am a terrible mother and responsible for her 'trauma'. She threatened to kill herself if I didn't agree to put her on testosterone and arrange 'top surgery'.

After much patience, persistence and luck we finally found a psychiatrist that Grace could work with. He prescribed anti-anxiety medication. It started to work. He also addressed the elephant in the room. Grace has Autism Spectrum Disorder (ASD). Most trans-identifying teenagers do.

Grace spent most of 2021 in a sad cycle of excitement at finding a new job and then despair at losing the job in the next lockdown. It put her deeper into a depression.

With the help of her psychiatrist, Grace slowly got better and weathered these storms. She returned to her first love of art. She drew and drew and drew. She created characters and a fantasy world and shared it with online friends.

Things were getting better. Slowly.

Until her younger sister Claire decided that she was trans too.

Like Grace, Claire is also mildly autistic. I do not like the term Autism Spectrum Disorder (ASD). The word 'disorder' sets my teeth on edge. I prefer the term 'neurodiverse'.

Neurodiverse females are vastly overrepresented in presentations of gender dysphoria. These girls already feel like aliens in human skin. They don't fit in anywhere.

The assertion that ASD is a disorder to be fixed, not a difference to be accepted has a direct parallel with the assertion that femininity is a flaw to be corrected, not a quiet power to be asserted.

Neurodiverse kids are prone to hyper-fixations. Grace was hyper-fixated on a gender transition. She believed it to be the cure to all her woes. Hyper-fixations take a while to pass, but pass they do.

Perhaps Grace's trans-identity exploration is an attempt to escape the 'tism' of her own biologically defined nature. Binary – zeros and ones – male and female – black and white. She knows instinctively that only the surface of existence is binary. The deeper layers of mystery are spectrums, categories, classifications, associations, affinities and affiliations.

Identity is a complex set of layers. And each layer is constructed differently.

It is my heart-felt belief that my dear daughter Grace is not actually trans. She is just gay and has applied the binary logic so inherent to her genetic makeup – 'I like women, therefore I am a man'.

And Claire idolises her older sister. This is peer contagion at its most pernicious.

Covid placed impossible stresses on our health care system and our communities. Covid damaged businesses, supply lines, and our children's sense of security.

Grace's mental health crisis had been brewing for years. When she turned thirteen, we took her to a few psychologists who all nodded and listened and reassured me that there was nothing terribly wrong with her. She was just a sensitive child who lacked resilience. The psychologists never consider autism as a possible cause of her anxiety.

I can recall moments of acute anxiety at a similar age. I remember sitting alone in the house and picking up the phone, dialling random numbers and asking strangers to help me. But I didn't know what was wrong.

The pressure to bottle it up, to cope, and to pretend to be a normal human being was actually perversely helpful. It pointed me in a direction.

When Grace was finally able to see a psychiatrist, he was at pains to explain that he is not a gender specialist and repeatedly tried to refer me to a Gender Clinic. I refused to be palmed off and he started unravelling the riddle that is Grace.

She has been doing so much better under his generalised, not specialised, psychiatric care.

He has helped me understand the many layers of this modern mania of trans-genderism.

Exposure to porn at a young age is a common trigger for a deep fear of sexual assault.

When Grace was growing up, I did not install porn blockers or other parental software controls. I took a libertine attitude thinking that being the canny little kid she was, she would work out how to bypass the controls soon enough and resent me heavily for them. I kept the computers in the lounge room and maintained as close an eye as I could while respecting her privacy. More fool me.

What I did not understand was the step up in the availability and perversity of porn that is commonly available.

My advice to other parents in this situation is to restrict your daughter's unsupervised computer and device time. She will hate you for it. And it is very difficult to enforce. But ready access to highly demeaning porn is traumatising. One of Grace's underlying motivations to seek a gender transition was not wanting to be on the receiving end of 'that'.

Another layer is anxiety.

"I can't see myself being nineteen," said Grace just after her eighteenth birthday. She could not see a future for herself. For the world. The world outside her door looked so bad to her.

This is the same anxiety that previous generations have faced. But for Grace, everything was worsened by the fears that Covid would trigger an apocalypse.

The most distressing element of Grace's mental health journey was when she made a false accusation of abuse against my husband to her psychiatrist. I know this accusation is false because I was in the room at the time.

Grace was about eleven and I honestly cannot remember what started it all. She was hysterical and my husband picked her up, put her in a chair, held her there and maintained direct eye contact while shouting at her.

A distressing childhood memory but hardly abuse.

Grace declared that this event was the 'trauma' that had triggered her and caused her to become trans.

Teenage girls are famous for self-absorption. Most of them mature through it. Their self-perception is slowly tempered by reality. They come to realise that much of what has gone wrong in their lives is the consequence of their own actions, and their need for validation settles down as their surety of self improves.

There are many layers to this modern phenomenon of huge numbers of teenagers identifying as trans. Peer contagion, self-loathing, neurodiversity, fear of sexual assault, anxiety, body issues, online toxicity, hero worship and narcissism are just the elements that I have been able to discern from my own two daughters.

But there is hope.

Grace is now nearly 21. She has come full circle and is now identifying as 'gender-fluid'. And quite frankly, I can live with that.

Claire is 17, and still deeply captured by trans-ideology.

I nearly lost her when her school guidance officer and school nurse, following official advice from their respective state departments encouraged Claire's brand-new gender identity. They told her that because we do not 'affirm' her, this means we are being abusive. They further goaded her into declaring herself a 'mature minor', so the school nurse could give her a referral to a gender clinic. Again, they were following official advice from radical activists who have infiltrated the state education and state health departments.

Luckily, we got wind of the situation from Grace and we intervened before Social Services got involved.

Today, my daughters both still live at home and our truce has mellowed into a fragile peace.

How has this happened? I've had lots of time to think this through, and I put it down to love, forgiveness and boundaries.

A child targeted by activists spreading radical gender theory is fed many lies.

"You were born in the wrong body. That's why you feel so wrong, weird, and out of place."

"You need to take testosterone and have top surgery to live an authentic life."

"Don't tell your parents about this. They won't understand. They will be angry and ashamed of you. They will throw you out of the house."

And on and on it goes.

An inescapable cycle of exploiting the turmoil of adolescence to create a false divide between loving parents and despairing children. An insidious mantra of estrangement that paints parents as cruel monsters who refuse to understand.

Social media, friendship groups, and even in the classroom. They cannot escape this mantra that the reason for all their many woes is that they are 'trans'. And the 'cure' is puberty blockers, testosterone injections and 'top surgery'.

I have come to firmly believe that love is the only cure.

Reassure your daughter that you love her and that you are her ally in this fight.

Spend dedicated time with her.

Grace and I have committed to a movie date once a week. We have seen some gems and some bombs and love dissecting the plots and characterization. This time spent together is slowly repairing our mother-daughter relationship.

I take Claire out to have sushi together once a week. Creating a 'safe space' where she can tell me anything that is on her mind. We still have a long way to go. But I am confident that we can get there.

But not without forgiveness.

A child in the grips of an induced gender identity crisis is in acute psychic distress. She has been convinced that there is a 'cure' for her many woes, but you – her mother – are withholding it.

I don't deserve the horrible words that have been flung at me by both my daughters. My husband does not deserve the false accusations of abuse.

I forgive them. Because I understand the omni-presence of radical gender theory in their lives. And I remember enough of my teenage self to realise that I would have fallen for it too.

Forgiveness for these coached insults and horrible lies is the only way forward. Anxiety adds a distinct tone to a distressed child's voice. I learned to listen for it and tempered my reaction, even though I know I was coming across as a stone-cold bitch.

The trifecta of this puzzle is boundaries.

Activists are pushing a narrative that failing to affirm a child's brand-new gender identity constitutes child abuse. This narrative is being used as grounds by trans-activists (who have infiltrated Social Services) to seize confused children from loving homes.

And so, unfortunately, you must minimally affirm your daughter lest you lose her entirely.

I use my daughters' chosen names when addressing them and do my best with the linguistic gymnastics that are their chosen pronouns. In return, my daughters have agreed not to pursue chemical or surgical gender transition whilst living at home.

These boundaries take away the grounds for the State to seize them. They concede enough ground to my daughters to keep them safe, and give them time to think.

Once again, self-appointed experts working for the State are deeming mothers 'unfit' and seizing their children.

Please help us keep our kids safe from harm. Radical gender theory confers no benefits on vulnerable children and poses huge risks to their mental health.

CHAPTER 4

Melinda's story

Husband

I had my counsellor's hat on. It seemed to be the only way I could deal with the things I was hearing that were coming out of my husband's mouth. He had been my lovely redheaded childhood sweetheart since I was 15 years old and he 16. I could feel my heart becoming bruised with each word. To this day, there is still a part that is the colour purple despite all the healing that has taken place over the last 10 plus years.

For what seemed like years, I listened while he fought the thoughts in his head, and the impact they were having on him. During those months, all I remember are the words 'become a eunuch', 'surgery', 'no sex anymore', 'transgender' and 'a new name'. I wondered what these words and phrases meant, and what to do with the fog of confusion that was beginning to cloud my mind and my heart.

As I write, I feel physically ill at the memories of this time, of our home, the church we attended, my job and our family. These all became lost to me because of this one decision of his.

It seemed like overnight, he transformed from male to female. In reality it has been a process that has taken years, way before our conversations began. I was slowly realising that my beautiful husband was not who he said he was. He was not who everyone else thought he was. Marriage and children were just a façade that he had put on.

I remember a man who whistled for his family as he came home from work, loved to bike ride, invest in marginalised men, sang to 'Art and Garfunkel' with a beautiful voice. And had the most beautiful smile. Today, my heart hurts for him. He is someone who is trying to find himself in a false identity. As far as I know, he is not happy, or settled within himself. He suffers anxiety and other mental health issues. I've watched first hand as transgender ideology wreaks havoc on people's lives.

I'm trying to remember the sequence of events, but I can't; all I remember are the feelings. One day, I had a husband, the next, I had one who was growing his hair long, picking women's clothes up off the side of the road, and watching transgender porn in those clothes after I had gone to bed. I wonder not if he did, but for how long he had been wearing my skirts when I was out. Maybe it is why I feel uncomfortable wearing skirts and dresses now.

Before he started talking about transgender, I had been doing a unit at college on this exact topic while studying for my Masters in Counselling. Something about the issues discussed seemed very familiar, but I didn't know why. God was preparing me for what was to come. I wasn't prepared for being marginalised or condemned by my family because I wasn't prepared to go along with this new construct he thought he was, and that he had created.

It took about six months before the counsellor's hat of protection began to slip off my head. When it did, it fell with a great thud leaving the mum and wife that I was vulnerable to the danger I felt I was in. My eyes were now on my girls, my family and my marriage. What did all this mean for us? No counselling training or experience helped here.

As my husband's voice of transgender became louder, my voice of truth was silenced. I became so confused, and felt protective over our children. I started to worry they were not safe. The issue had nothing to do with their physical safety, but rather their emotional and mental safety – they were 9 and 12 at the time. I felt helpless to protect them from a father and a world that believed a lie and is lost. I felt we had been betrayed by the same man I had stood at the altar with who had promised me leadership and protection. Now I was in a position of trying to emotionally protect myself and my children from my husband and their own dad.

This whole journey led to much counselling that never seemed to go anywhere. I felt caught in a web of lies and deceit. I tried so hard to understand and accept this new story, but I knew it was a lie. I could not settle and I realised I had to make the choice. I packed the car with our children and very few possessions, and moved temporarily into a friend's converted double garage down the road. Years later in my own rental, my husband came to drop something off to me. I saw my childhood sweetheart, long grey hair, black handbag, jeans, frilly pink top, but still *him*. I rooted myself firmly to the ground. Every part of me wanted to sink into his body, feel his arms around me, smell his familiar smell and hear his familiar voice. My head was so confused. The person standing in front of me was not him anymore, it was someone else. It was him but it wasn't. His voice sounded higher, there was fat in places that would only be fat on a female from the oestrogen pills, and his skin was smooth from the electrolysis. He appeared so unhappy and so awkward and I could sense his desperate need for acceptance. The only thing familiar was the tender look he gave me, that familiar look of love. The person I had known for twenty years had disappeared. I can only explain this transition from my perspective as 'having a family member die or go missing, and no body to bury'.

From the moment the conversations began on his transgender identity, my femininity, womanhood and mothering role felt threatened. I felt dirty, a fake, as if I had all of a sudden become non-existent and obliterated. I wondered who I was now and where I fit in the world and with other females. There have been a few dear friends who have supported me in the best way they know how. As a whole people either gave their opinion, ignored our story by either changing the subject or physically turning away, didn't ask if I or the girls were ok, how this was affecting us or if they could do anything to support us. There were those who were quick to blame me, "it must be your fault for not being a good wife". The most ignorant response was, 'if you stayed, you would be a lesbian'. I was still me. He had changed, not me.

While we can only say so much or offer limited support on an issue as messy as transgender in families when we ourselves have not been in the same arena, we can listen to understand. We judge, fail to offer support or listen when we ourselves are threatened by things we don't understand or accept. As a culture, we need to realise that our identity doesn't need to be threatened just because of someone's story.

Daughters

We named her after my great aunt. Her name means shining light. She is my firstborn, so beautiful, chubby and healthy. It was at the time she was put to my face that I knew she was not a neurotypical child, but one with a precious and unique way of looking at life from inside her own bubble. There was something in those newly opened eyes that stared right into me. At the same time, there was something in her body that did not want to or did not know how to connect with mine. This is the way our relationship continued, both of us seeing and knowing each other deeply, yet struggling to connect. When she was 12, my suspicions throughout her life were confirmed, with a diagnosis of autism.

It was when she was 7, at the age when children are becoming more aware of those around them, their separateness from family, and awareness of themselves, that I was not shaken when she said to her dad and I, "I wish I was a boy". She did not say, "I am a boy". Two very different constructs. My response, "Do you darling?". Her dad's response was silence. Later on in my marriage, I would discover why. She expressed nothing more of her statement until she was in her late teens. As a result of autism my daughter did not talk a lot or engage in many conversations. This increased as she became older.

Throughout her childhood and into her teens, my daughter appeared to prefer her own company to that of others, and any play was parallel and concrete, not imaginary. We could be at a playgroup, and there she would be, sitting with all the books, back turned away from the other children in her own bubble. Books, pencils, paper, matchbox cars, blocks and later on technology became her playmates, and her younger sister under duress. She seemed not to be interested in others, and as she became older, humoured their intellect compared to her own. All aspects of autism, not transgender. I had a young child, now a young adult trying to fit herself into a world that she doesn't relate to and that doesn't relate to her unique way of looking at the world. The choice for her, as is the choice for all of us in life, is to change to fit into the world we live within, or follow our own God created uniqueness.

From that statement at 7 years old, the physical changes began. It began with no longer wanting to wear dresses, then no frills on tops, baggy clothes, loose tops and only pants, removal of her earrings, cutting her hair short at 15. I pushed aside the thought that maybe the outward change was a sign that bigger things were to come. The emotional changes were not as clear. My daughter was not a big talker and appeared to prefer her own company. I did not really know what was going on inside for her. I even took her shopping for the clothes she preferred, boy tops, boy shorts, boot leg pants. My motto as a parent was, 'Which mountains do I climb, and which battles do I fight?'. To me, which clothes my daughter chose were just a preference for comfort, just as blocks and cars were her choice of play.

I'm sure there were other signs that my daughter wished to change her identity, but I was going through my own trauma. By this time, I had separated from my children's father, and he was going through the process of changing sexes. I tried to protect my children from false thinking and lies, while having to send them to the place where the lies came from. I didn't quite know what to think of the gender fluidity ideology that our society was embracing despite having a Master's degree in counselling and studying gender dysphoria. I didn't know what to say to my children regarding their dad; after all he loved them. How was I to voice what I thought the truth to be without pointing a condemning finger at their dad?

Conversation with my daughter was short and to the point, just like the day she told me she was non-binary. I knew what it was, but I wanted to hear if she knew and why. I did not know what to say when one day at around 16, she came home with a binder to flatten her chest that her dad had helped her buy. It seemed that the more she found her voice in her outward presentation, the more I lost mine as a parent, and felt silenced. I told her that her body was beautiful just the way it was, and offered to wash it for her. Inside I was crying and screaming, wanting to hide my child away and protect her from lies, danger and a grey fog of identity confusion that was coming for her. Unconsciously, I knew that if I spoke the truth and tried to protect her, I would lose my child. I was just putting off the inevitable.

I wonder how my eldest daughter's changes have affected her younger sister. What does she think? She would push me for my opinion, ready to pounce verbally if she didn't like what I said. It seemed nothing was quite right. She tested me by wanting to call our female kitten by a masculine name. I felt helpless to protect her as well. At home mum said one thing, at school, with friends and with dad, other beliefs were heard. I was in a losing battle for my children. If I spoke up more or louder, would they have heard or believed me? My hunch was that the inevitable loss of my children would have come sooner.

I have never heard my daughter tell me she was transgender, I only see it by the testosterone she takes daily, the lowering of her voice, the protruding voice box, the muscles on her shoulders mixed with feminine softness, the angular jaw line and the removal of her breasts. That last one makes me feel ill and want to scream. I felt (and still feel) powerless to protect my own child from the world, her father and now a boyfriend. A child with ASD who takes on the characteristics and identities of others in her influence, not really understanding or being aware of the long-term consequences of such a choice.

The last I saw or heard from my eldest daughter was five years ago. I thought that her visit to stay with me was an opportunity to finally share my concerns, identify truth, her value and above all my love for her. All I can think is, 'it is my job as a mum to speak truth and life into her'. I was losing my child, quickly. Let's say, it did not go well. Maybe all she heard was judgement and non-acceptance. That's the message our world gives right. 'If you don't accept my 'true' identity, you don't accept me'. No, I will not accept the perceived change in identity, but I do accept, and fiercely love my child. My arms will always be open, and I will always be waiting for her whether it is as the female that I birthed, or the perceived male she has constructed within herself. She is my child, God's child and very much loved.

CHAPTER 5

Rachel's story

I have an 18 year old daughter identifying as "Trans". She has changed her name at school, among her friends, peers and teachers and now our extended family. She is now in the midst of Year 12 and her HSC.

Elise "identifies" as Elijah-Eli for short-a trans boy/man. We call her E. She corrects us if we misgender her but gives us a pass if we self correct – it's infuriating and humiliating.

Her Dad and I are devastated as we had no warning and no idea. Her older sister and her sister's boyfriend knew before we did, as did all her friends and the school.

I have been on an emotional rollercoaster now for some months and I've engaged a psychologist for myself because I was beginning to get very depressed and was having some dark thoughts.

The Principal of her school is a wonderful woman and she and I have had a meeting to discuss E. She apologised that the school hadn't informed us of E's "school transition" as she was unaware that we didn't know. She told me the Transgender issue with students has been shockingly sudden and they have had no professional reports, information or guidance made available from the Education Department or anywhere else as to how they need to proceed other than to nurture each student as an individual as they normally would.

E is a very good student, a talented singer, performer and writer who has trained with NIDA's Young Actors Studio and is interested in attending VCA (Victorian College of the Arts) next year. She is Performing Arts Captain and a prefect and is on the Student Executive at her private girls school in Sydney. Her Principal holds her in very high esteem.

"E" is also very well versed in trans ideology and knows what to say to therapists to convince them of her belief that she is really a boy. Her Dad and I organised an appointment including E with a psychologist at "YouTherapy", a practice in Crows Nest which I found online and which had an interest in youth care. During the appointment we were able to express to her and E our deep misgivings about testosterone treatment and surgery and wanting her to delay at least until after she has completed her HSC, hoping to buy time for her "to come to her senses" but she turned on a very convincing performance for the therapist that we just don't understand how she is so distressed about her "unmanly" voice among other things, that she has begun to hate having singing lessons and has asked her singing coach to work at helping her to deepen her voice!

As parents we felt we were able to express our feelings and the therapist acknowledged that and suggested to E that maybe she could think about delaying transition until she finished Year 12 as she obviously has very loving and supportive parents who are very worried about how this will affect her.

E started to cry and said, "they just don't understand how I feel and how horrible it is for me!"

Again, we were at a loss as to what to say or do.

We decided not to see that therapist again as she sent me a follow up email and included some contacts for vocal coaches for E. I guess she meant well but I was stunned! She was obviously a Gender Affirming clinician and I hadn't spotted it!

I'm wiser now but E has since seen our GP who has referred her to Clinic 16 in St Leonards (a gender "health" clinic) who she had a "Telehealth call" with. Unbeknown to her and "Clifton" I listened in on the call and typed up a transcript on my phone because I'm going to document everything for the future.

My daughter was really happy and upbeat and joking with the guy? - sounded like a man. He asked her when she started feeling like she was "trans" and as per the "script" she said "Oh I can remember back in primary school (co-ed primary by the way) when my friends and I played families I always played the Dad role!" (Really? Who hasn't done that before? I was George Harrison when my 3 brothers and I pretended we were the Beatles in our backyard!) I played footy and cricket with my brothers and was known as "Tom" (as in tomboy) for a while. I thought it was fun but I never thought I was actually a boy!

Anyway she claimed she "came out" to one friend in Year 7 and had been "gender fluid" since she was 13 and thought she was lesbian for a while which she apparently realised was sooo wrong! (I hate to say it but she had a friend in the year above her at the time who also claimed she was lesbian and E does tend to copy others unfortunately so we took that with a grain of salt).

She also claimed she came out at school as "Trans" in year 10 although she didn't come out to us until the end of year 11 which was last year.

E also clearly stated to him she had read all about it on You Tube!

They continued the telecall with him asking her about us and what we thought.

"Well because they don't understand they have been seeking out information online and have been getting their info from conservatives like Jordan Peterson, Matt Walsh and Ben Shapiro-they're being brainwashed!"

Apparently this was very funny because they both laughed and scoffed at our obvious ignorance!

My husband has spoken to work colleagues who are also dealing with this in their families, and some of our family members who are physicians and a cousin who is a gay man.

I have researched multiple sources including authors like Helen Joyce who has written "TRANS", Abigail Shrier "Irreversible Damage" - Teenage Girls and the Transgender Craze, Dr Gordon Neufeld "Hold on to your Kids" and I'm on a waiting list for the release of Dr Miriam Grossman's new book "Lost in Trans Nation-a Child Psychologist's Guide out of the Madness" I have also watched a lot of podcasts for example "Gender through a Wider Lens" among many others and many interviews, with detransitioners.

I'm far from ignorant or ill-informed.

The call continued with him talking her through the process to get her started on testosterone. She's booked in for blood tests at the clinic in a few months and he doesn't anticipate any problems because she is 18 and young and healthy (the irony of that comment was flabbergasting).

This was all on the phone which means that Clifton has never met her in person. He didn't ask for her medical history. I told her to tell him she has an inherited blood clotting disorder. She did so, and he replied, "Oh that shouldn't be a problem like you're 18!" "We'll put you on a "gentler" dose of testosterone because you're doing HSC SO AS NOT TO CAUSE ANY PROBLEMS! Higher doses are sometimes an issue!"

I didn't need anyone to tell me that - obviously they can be an issue, because she is a girl!

E was previously diagnosed a couple of years ago by a psychiatrist at the Gordon Clinic as having ADHD and generalised anxiety and she was prescribed Ritalin. No mention was made of transgenderism by her or the doctor (it wasn't a fad back then!).

Mind you my daughter didn't actually ask Clifton from Clinic 16 if he's a doctor, nurse, endocrinologist, counsellor, psychologist, GP, nothing. I went onto the Clinic 16 website to find out who he is and no practitioners are listed. I found the Medical Director who runs the clinic on LinkedIn!!

E asked me to attend her psychologist appointment that week (because the psychologist would like to talk to me too.) I knew that because I had emailed her previously (E is supposed to see her twice and get her to write a "report" to bring back to the clinic. Thanks Clifton!).

I don't hold out much hope that she will be diagnosed with anything other than gender dysphoria by this psychologist because she uses the WPATH SOC 8 - World Professional Association of Transgender Health Standards of Care Version 8. Released in 2022 - If you haven't already looked into this Association and their history please do, it is horrifying. Check out the new section in Version 8 on Eunuchs- that's men who identify as eunuchs and want their testicles and sometimes also their penis's removed to affirm their identity- I know this psychologist uses this Association's protocols because I emailed her and asked.

So you can see what's happening here. These clinicians and doctors are all on the same page ie: medically transition anyone who asks especially if they're young and healthy. I don't understand the underlying reasoning because it doesn't make sense. It's just unconscionable and quite frankly exhausting.

CHAPTER 6
Emma and Paul's story

The end of August 2018 marked a significant turning point in our family's life. Our daughter, on the cusp of 14, crossed paths with Charlie, a new student at her school. Drawn together by a shared affinity for the French language, they quickly formed a connection. Little did we know, Charlie's influence would usher in a series of transformations in our daughter's life.

Charlie, identifying as a trans boy, played a pivotal role in our daughter's journey, encouraging her to cope with stress through self-harm. Swift intervention from the school however, spared her from further harm – to a certain extent, given that they were very affirming of her gender dysphoria – as she found herself under the care of the local Child and Adolescent Mental Health Services team.

In the aftermath, our daughter's demeanour underwent a seismic shift. Once a girl who embraced her femininity, she now adorned baggy, dark clothing, erecting a barrier between herself and the world. Communication dwindled, replaced by a palpable withdrawal. Even the warmth of a mother's kiss, once cherished, became an unwelcome intrusion.

By mid-December, just over three months later, our daughter emerged from her cocoon, revealing a complex identity—polysexual non-binary masculine. Renaming herself Jessie, she expressed a desire to shed the physical remnants of her femininity, citing a lifelong discomfort with her breasts. This revelation blindsided us, as she had never hinted at such feelings before, not even during the onset of puberty.

Charlie, an avid researcher on matters of identity, became a guiding force. Christmas brought a note from her, signed "Dad," affirming pride in our daughter's newfound self. In this evolving narrative, Charlie assumed the role of "Mum" for another friend in their trans circle.

Navigating our daughter's identity became a labyrinth of terms and pronouns. While she accepted the title of "daughter" at home, outside, the world knew her as Jessie. Tensions arose between her desire for acceptance and our grounding in familiarity.

Recent revelations brought a glimmer of hope. In a vulnerable moment, our daughter opened up to me, her mother, embracing the validating approach. She expressed a wish for a name change and different pronouns. A delicate negotiation followed, revealing the intricate dance between acceptance and understanding.

In the wake of her evolving identity, our daughter pursued changes at school—officialising her name, donning the boys' uniform, and exploring binders, a journey met with mixed reactions. Conversations hinted at a future marked by breast reduction fundraisers and hormonal treatments, amplifying the complexity of her path.

As the digital realm became a lifeline, our once-strict rules on internet usage evolved. Yet, this newfound freedom proved a double-edged sword, magnifying her struggles and fostering an environment where her issues loomed larger than life.

Reflecting on her past, she unearthed a history of childhood bullying, the echoes of which manifested in social anxiety. This journey, laden with emotional highs and lows, delved into self-perception, body image, and the quest for self-discovery. The spectre of sleep troubles and disordered eating emerged, each thread weaving into the intricate tapestry of our daughter's identity.

To assist our daughter, it took us a year to find a psychologist who would focus on exploration rather than mainstream affirmation approach (difficult to find as vilified by the masses); it was like finding a golden nugget. We don't know how we would have carried on without her help as we were about to give in to peer pressure, and we are so grateful for her.

Amidst these complexities, a decision loomed on the horizon—an exchange program to France, a quest for self-exploration in a familiar yet foreign landscape. But even here, the tendrils of gender identity extended, posing challenges in the pursuit of a life-changing opportunity.

The decision was made, she could go to France on the condition she stopped self-harming. She agreed.

The time apart provided much needed respite for everyone. The internet made it difficult to completely remove her from bad influences, but having the physical and geographical separation was helpful.

Then Covid hit.

Our daughter had the opportunity to return but she decided to stick it out with her host family, who were happy to have her stay. The restrictions in France were tough. The communities were locked down and our daughter had to carry a note if she went out. Life wasn't much different for her there though to be honest. She had voluntarily locked herself down prior to Covid by secluding herself in her bedroom with the curtains closed, always on her mobile phone.

During her time in France, she realised she was actually fed up with the internet and missing social interactions. That was a big surprise to us! It was the forced lock down that made her realise there is more to life and she was missing out.

Four months after returning to Australia our daughter finally opened up to me, her mother. One morning, she poured out her heart and confessed she had no good memories from growing up. She blamed us, her parents, for every bad thing she could remember. She had been bullied at school and wanted to escape herself. For hours she recalled memory after memory with pain and sorrow. And that now as a result she is suffering from PTSD, social anxiety, and a myriad of other mental illnesses.

As painful as it was, it opened a way for us to share our concerns. As her mother I shared about the discoveries I had been making online. Tragic story after tragic story of people who had undergone transitioning treatments, only to be left devastated and permanently scarred. We assured her that her sexual orientation would not harm her, but attempting to change her identity to a male would leave her irreversibly damaged.

She was still insisting she was male but didn't take any further steps to medicalise her identity even though she was considering a double mastectomy. She was very dismissive of detransitioners who 'should have known better and were not as sure as she was'.

Then, one day out of the blue, she came to me and asked if I had kept one of her favourite black lacy tops. I was momentarily stunned before revealing to her I had kept many of her clothes.

We began pulling out dresses and reminiscing and she was happy. It was all I could do not to jump and twirl and shout, I couldn't believe it! Was my little girl coming back to me?

I didn't hound her or ask her any questions. We gave her all the space and time she needed to figure herself out. She gradually began wearing more feminine clothing and choosing to embrace the truth she is female regardless of what she wears or how she feels about herself.

Our daughter is seeing her fourth psychologist and addressing the underlying issues and diagnosing all her mental health challenges. She still has high levels of stress and anxiety, but it is nothing compared to how stressed and anxious she was when identifying as male.

Her journey has been so hard on the whole family. Her two younger brothers have been very confused through it all. She didn't want any affection; no hugs or kisses, and that was really hard for me as her mother (nearly 6 years without a kiss or a cuddle, and still counting). While there is still pain and sorrow, there is now great hope as our daughter works on self-acceptance. We hope that one day she will fully reconcile with us and recognise the journey she and we have been through.

We felt so alone, so isolated through it all. It is so important to hang in there and to be strong.

We want to encourage other families to never give up hope.

We lost friends and had no one to talk to. It was such a lonely time. We felt as if the world was against us, especially the healthcare and school systems. We felt terribly misunderstood.

It was so hard to watch our daughter hate herself and deny who she is. It was terribly painful to accept how she felt about herself, about us.

It is so important to have boundaries and to say things like, "maybe this is how you feel, but I don't feel that way and I'm really concerned for you, for your wellbeing" or "this may be your journey, this is not your siblings' and you need to leave them out of it" when she started indoctrinating them.

We discovered other families going through the same difficulties. We connected with other parents in similar situations. We found a practitioner who addresses the underlying issues and does not just affirm her confusion and pain.

There is definitely light at the end of the tunnel. Easier said than done but just don't give up.

One analogy that sustained us is that as parents, we are a lighthouse, strong like a rock, firm on the ground and not get drowned with them. The light gives direction and acts as a warning to steer clear of danger. We need to be that for our children.

During the darkest time we also rediscovered our faith. We found great comfort and hope in the church and in God. It gave us hope and meaning and is helping us as we continue to heal as individuals and as a family.

CHAPTER 7

Danielle's story

I have three children. My eldest is my daughter, Emily, who is now 31 years old, and two younger sons, Joshua and William.

It's been quite a journey since Emily disclosed to me, when she was still a teenager, that she thought she had been born in the wrong body.

She was born a beautiful little girl, and she now feels that she is a male.

Her dad, my former partner, would take her to the shops when she was little and let her buy whatever she wanted. I have since learned that he bought her boy clothes and let herself be called Sean. I didn't know that he was validating her identity as a boy. In my mind, this is where it all started.

When my daughter was five years old, I took her to our GP after she told me she didn't want a pair of lips, and would compulsively peel them. She told me she was scared of footsteps and soft toys. I got a referral to a psychologist who said that both she and her younger brother were exhibiting sexualised behaviours.

This seemed to confirm my previous suspicions that my daughter had been sexually abused by her father.

My ex partner took me to Family Court to try and prove that he didn't sexually abuse Emily and Josh. The fight took ten years, as I fought for custody of my children and for the truth. In the end, I lost all three children, after they were ordered by the Court to live with my ex-partner full time. This was devastating for me. In spite of the Court ruling, I have endeavoured to remain in close contact with all of my children.

When Emily was a teenager, she visited a GP to try and help her with certain issues she was dealing with. The GP referred her to a psychiatrist, who started her on hormone therapy. I was shocked when I took her to her appointment and saw the patients in the waiting room, who had or were undergoing gender transitions. I objected to my daughter receiving this 'treatment' when she hadn't even had a psychological assessment, but I was overruled. I strongly felt that my daughter needed counselling, not help to transition to become a male. I felt so angry at this doctor, who I felt was robbing my daughter of a future chance to become a mother and a wife. I made a complaint to the medical board about this doctor, but nothing was done.

I have grieved my own chance at becoming a grandmother to any children my daughter might have had.

I stayed in contact with Emily throughout this period when she started hormone therapy, despite my strong objections. She told me once that she felt she was dying. I told her I thought she needed to stop this dangerous therapy. She told me she had had kidney failure twice since starting on the course of hormone therapy. She has never in her life had kidney problems before this. I spoke to her on a number of occasions and pleaded with her to stop what she was doing. I was worried it would kill her and I told her that. She ended up in the Royal Adelaide Hospital twice. I visited her there. It was very painful to me as a mother to see my daughter taking this route. I tried to reach out and speak the truth to her.

I had a regular relationship with Emily until she got involved with a girl who I think has a narcissistic personality disorder. She convinced Emily to block all contact with me. She isolated her from her own mother. It definitely feels like she is in a domestic violence situation in this current relationship.

As a result, I haven't been in contact with Emily since October 2022.

A year later, her brother Joshua texted me to say that unless I accepted and respected Emily's decision to become a male, he would stop all contact with me as well. That has also broken my heart. He has recently had a child with his partner, and it means that I've also lost contact with my granddaughter, who I have only ever met once. The ripple effect that this issue has had on our family has been devastating.

All along, I have stood for truth, and in particular the truth that she is a girl; she was born a girl, and she will always be a girl, no matter what. I love my children more than they will ever know but I cannot accept that my daughter is a male and I fear what this treatment and course that she has chosen will mean for her in the future.

CHAPTER 8

Kelly's story

Our story is still going on, and there are many unanswered questions.

We don't know where this journey will end, so I have not included any names or sexes of the people involved, but in essence, it is about our precious, much-loved adult married child not being happy as the person God created them to be.

It is also about a very little child (our grandchild) thrust into the middle of concepts they have no way of processing or even questioning.

It is also about us as parents who have been silenced and can't speak life or truth into any of their lives and who desperately don't want to lose our child or their beautiful family.

In mid 2022, we started hearing a few things from our young grandchild that did not make sense. There was a time when they had to stay with us because of COVID-19, and the child's parents sent some very questionable stuff for us to share with the child. They would have known that my husband and I would not appreciate it or share it. Looking back, I can see that my child would have known that the information they sent would get this Christian parent asking questions; it probably worked more quickly than they expected.

Over the next few weeks, a few more incidents got me questioning exactly what was happening in this family's home. As I spent time with and talked to my grandchild at this stage, I was correcting and disputing things being said, telling them about correct biology and gender, assuring the child that God did not make mistakes.

At the time, I was going through a medical procedure. A few days before I went into the hospital for the next part of my treatment, I found out that my child was not only questioning their sexuality but that, in private and online, had changed their name and the gender they identify as.

We were not told anything directly; we just started hearing things. In the end, I had to approach them and start the conversation. During this conversation, I was put on notice that there would come a day when we would be unable to acknowledge this child I had loved, encouraged and looked after by using the name we had lovingly given them.

I was told a few things in this conversation that I saw as trauma points or at least contributing factors to the discontentment with who they are. Nothing terrible, but still a mounting level of trauma that would make anyone unhappy with or unsure of who they were supposed to be.

I was assured that a "professional" had been talking to them and they saw no trauma in their past; they were trans (can't think of the medical name) and should make the change. After speaking with my child, I heard enough to question and wanted to scream about all the trauma points I saw in that conversation.

All we felt that we could do is to pray. I felt like we were told in that moment that we would have to kill our child, the person we loved and raised. We had failed them as parents, and my heart was broken. Hopelessness threatened to engulf me. As Christians, all we could do was pray and trust God in the mess; after all, the decision is our child's to make, and all that is left for us to do is to live with the consequences.

We felt alone and did not know where to look; there is so much in the media about just accepting and embracing this with no thought for anyone else involved. If you question anything at all, you are labelled transphobic, and an awful, uncaring, judgemental person.

In the end, I am just a parent who wants their child back.

Before the Covid lockdowns, my child and I had spent a bit of time talking about their dreams and the steps they wanted to take to step into them.

But in the isolation of the lockdowns, this precious couple started to explore transgender ideology with no real questions from anyone else. I want to rescue them from this journey, from the deception that is engulfing them, the pain that is being caused for not just their household but their families that love them. I wish I had been more insightful and bold in the earlier part of this journey or that our relationship was stronger, so they would have felt comfortable confiding in me. I wish I had instilled in them the belief they were amazing as the person God created them to be, but today I am left feeling like I failed them in so many ways.

Since that initial conversation, there have been two conversations on the topic.

The major one came after I corrected a lie my grandchild was sprouting as fact. The next day, I was reprimanded for making the parents out to be lying to their child about women and men and which body parts belong to which gender. We were banned from seeing our grandchild for a few weeks.

So often, this beautiful child has been used as a pawn, and honestly, this is an added level of complexity and hurt to the whole situation. Our grandchild has been burdened with the task of alerting people about their parent's gender change; or at the very least, hinting about things changing. When I think about my grandchild, my heart aches so much. Before anything was said to any grandparent, the way they referred to this parent was changed, and they would correct us, saying, I don't have a ... I have two …. now.

Because we did not know what was going on, we were correcting them about biological facts, without realising we were causing more confusion. During a very honest conversation with my child, I was able to share how this affected me, that being asked to murder my living child was unfair and painful. Not being able to talk to my child about them because I only saw them as the person I loved, the person they were excited to be at the birth of this precious child and, of course, the child we raised.

I don't ever think I will be able to see them as anything other than the person they were born to be. I shared that it broke our hearts that the child we brought up was not happy with who they were created to be.

As a parent, having your child tell you that they are not happy with how they were created to be is crushing; the guilt, the heartache and the disappointment is something I wish on no other parents. As parents, we do our best, love our children, and try to encourage them. Yes, there were some stresses in our home growing up, and as a result, there were times of inconsistencies in parenting, but they were never not loved and always looked after.

At the time of writing this, we, the parents, are praying that God will give them (both spouses in that family) a fresh revelation of who they are created to be, that their eyes will be opened and that there will be a new confidence in all the amazing gifts and talents they have. We are also praying that they would grow to feel comfortable and confident again in their born gender. Both spouses have also declared faith in Jesus, so we have confidence that our prayers are worthwhile and not entirely in vain.

We love our child, their spouse and our grandchild, but having the threat hanging over us that there could be a day when a line is drawn in the sand, and changes enforced, weighs heavy like a millstone. I am still not sure if I will be able to cross that line in any form, and the very real consequence could be that we lose not only our child but their family and other family memories.

Watching your child go through this is heartbreaking, especially when there were no signs while they were growing up. As I said, we don't know what the future will bring, but today we are in a relationship with our child. They respond to their name, and we get to love them, but it is always with an air of fear that the line will be drawn, or that I will say something that they deem insulting or misgendering.

If the line is drawn and we can't cross it, the impact could split our family; we could lose not just one child, but at least another sibling because they have already told me I am wrong. As Christians, we will never stop praying for them; until that line is drawn, we have hope and rejoice in every chance we have to lavish them with love.

Are we navigating this time well? Probably not. We have a million questions and never seem to get any answers; we are hesitant to seek help because of the social pressure to accept the irreversible changes our child wants to make. We are worried that our thoughts and feelings will be dismissed and disregarded. For the time being, we are doing the best we can with our backs against the wall; we are trusting our loving Heavenly Father for a breakthrough.

Our greatest fear is that our family will become permanently divided.

I know those who are not Christian say that my reaction is all religious biases, but my heart's desire is for my kids to know that they were made in the image of a loving Heavenly Father, who as King David said "knit them together in my womb". I am a parent who has been told they made a child in confusion and that I failed to build them up in a way they could be confident in exactly who they are. I lovingly and diligently cared for this baby, I have prayed for good things for this child, we have helped them pick up the pieces when mistakes were made. Yet all I see today with this child is that I let them down and have not equipped them with the sense they need to recognise the lie.

Yes there is a large God element, but to be honest it is the crushed parent's heart that often takes me to my knees to pray for protection, revelation and grace for them…and myself.

CHAPTER 9
Natalie's story

Toothpaste in hot water does not make peppermint tea, like testosterone cannot make a woman into a man.

It is said, a fool vents all of his feelings, but the wise holds them back.

I have held my peace for so long and the suffering has not abated but become far worse. Try as I might, I have a very hard time being able to identify with the humanity of believing it's a good idea to chemically or surgically chop off sex body bits for mental health.

The time to speak has come.

I'm telling my story for the purpose of encouraging other parents and therapists in navigating the truth of the rapid onset of gender dysphoria (ROGD) trans phenomenon. This is something I feel both afraid to do because of the political climate, and something I feel I absolutely would regret not doing as a responsible parent.

I believe it is singularly the most profound event in all of culture that is deeply affecting families in our day.

We need to support each other with evidence-based medical and scientifically objective care, grace for what has been, wisdom from generations past and much courage for moving forward in the face of what is going to be proven to be a huge mistake.

In the interest of fairness, I, like many parents, have investigated the pro arguments of trans youth. These arguments all sound like the latest subculture at first blush, and easily dismissed as such. Nobody really cares what haircut or clothing choices youth individuate with. However, listen hard and long enough, and anyone concludes it's all incoherent and there is really no such thing as trans. To identify 'appearance' and 'preferences' of gender stereotypes as being 'trans' is disingenuous. Pop culture of the past century has never believed they were the opposite sex and never did they medicalise and threaten with self-harm in order to bully others into going along with such delusions. It is the lie that sex can be changed and the coercion to buy into this medicalised and quite frankly lethal fantasy that is at the heart of parental objections. Not hate, not bigotry, not phobia. Simply a concern for long term harm and a refusal to speak words we know aren't true. Objectively, it's personality disordered types that project accusations which are veiled confessions. Mirroring emotions that are intent to destroy or erase the self, are destined to also destroy or erase family relationships. Activists' tantrum, cancel and censor for the same reason an abuser does; the desire for power. Isn't it possible that the whole idea of a "trans" community is just a minority political party of individuals seeking power?

Our children are lent to us at best. We bring them into the world knowing that they will grow up, individuate and make their own lives. We hope they will choose a good life, with real values that optimise their health and success. If we're lucky, they include us in for the ride sometimes. Our hopes for them are not a desire for enmeshment on our part. They are the natural, selfless result of human bonding from birth.

When we see our teenagers making mistakes, we can either choose to control their every decision for fear of them getting hurt, or we can lovingly warn them of the potential dangers but allow them to make their own decisions even if things turn out for the worse, as an opportunity for them to grow up, with hopefully no long-term damage or high cost. Importantly we want to see them come to wisdom, reality and love on the terms of their Creator and not of ourselves. Loving them unconditionally doesn't mean enabling, but rather continuing to parent with boundaries and encouragement towards wholeness of health and success. For parents with teenagers and youth who have been captured by the Trans idea, the reality of parenting feels more like a hostage negotiation, and our children are not necessarily thriving.

There seems to have been a recent explosion in the awareness of narcissism as a label. It's true that everyone needs some healthy degree of self-interest or else we would not function in the world. That said, I wish someone had told me what someone with a Cluster B personality disorder looked like when I was young. It seems popular in the culture of which our children are immersed, that anyone can accuse anyone who does anything they don't like, of being a "total narcissist". Just another name to sling. The advice that goes along with what people have to do to deal with narcissism, to "Grey rock" and "Go no contact" is projected onto parents as if the shoe fits. What parents are suffering deeply with is called betrayal trauma. We see the game our children are trying to play and we know it's toxic. Like Inigo Montoya from the movie The Princess Bride, we hear you keep using those words, and we don't think it means what you think it means.

Just about every doctrine of the Transgender idea is grounded in mentally ill thinking. Love bombing, buying into shared fantasy, disregard for the rights of others, deceitfulness, manipulation for personal gain, a sense of being special, intense emotional outbursts and self-identity issues, self-harm, emptiness, sensitivity to perceived rejection, unstable one way relationships, projected accusations, only scratch the surface of the many dysfunctional behaviours. None of it fools anyone who isn't a people pleasing, codependent enabler. I should know, because once upon a time, I was the latter. All the years of therapy from the damage done by a Cluster B personality still doesn't prepare you for the reality of dealing with the extremely destructive influence of such a personality on our children's minds. It's a normal thing to individuate but to irreversibly exploit or be unaware of being exploited for want of fitting in with everything trendy and popular should never be acceptable. I believe many of our trans identified children are just high functioning autistic, creative, sensitive individuals who desperately want to fit in with their peers. Trans seems the perfect vehicle to protect from otherwise being bullied for the effects of trauma or autism. Thankfully, autistic people can not be Cluster B personalities and Cluster B personalities cannot be autistic, although the two types are like magnets until the autistic person wakes up.

Parents are being betrayed by clinicians, media, politicians, teachers and entertainment. I once heard a parent describe the trauma of watching their child transition as like being asked to watch your child, not just slowly die of cancer, but be expected to rejoice in it! To not use their "dead name" but to use the name of that selfish "murderer" that they want you to be besties with. In short, we find ourselves in a twilight zone of people we thought had our best interest at heart, feeding us ideas we know are excrement and telling us if we don't behave ourselves and smile sweetly, we will be killed off and "cancelled" too. We will not be dehumanised and demoralised by people we previously believed we could trust who have now made it very clear we cannot. Media, clinicians, teachers and even members of my own family have most certainly lost my trust forever. Their cowardice will be remembered for not standing up to the mentally deranged few who tell the world how grandiosely virtuous and oppressed they are while deliberately setting out to covertly undermine and abuse the nuclear family, parental bonds and wholesome religious authority with their own brand of gnostic pseudoscience. Parents are beyond angry for good reason.

Helen Joyce, author of the book Trans: When Ideology Meets Reality has said, parents who have gone along with everything their teens have demanded as "lifesaving health care", will fight to the death sooner than acknowledge they have irrevocably harmed their own children with a promise that had no evidence of ever being delivered. Reality tends to break denial over time. Just as the guards from the Russian gulags were haunted by the atrocities they committed by believing absurdities, to the point of their own suicides, so too will the parents of this generation of our most mentally and emotionally vulnerable.

If it's true that the extended family story is formative to understanding how we grow in our process of human development, I offer one mother's story in its brief entirety, to the vast ROGD tree. I hope this helps therapists to remember what they have forgotten, and gives them courage to change their tune before the inevitable tsunami of lawsuits arrive.

There may be many pathways that make our children vulnerable to the lie that they are born in the wrong body. My story is just one of thousands, yet I believe is a window into what sort of fertile ground had been unwittingly prepared for planting the seeds of my own daughter's mental suffering.

The name of my daughter has been changed.

Sometimes, family is the dearest thing to your heart because your heart has a hole in it where a missing parent should have been. For me it was my dad. The 1960s and 70s was a decade of free love that saw legalised breaking of family structures. It was a culture sold as freedom, but in my opinion, the ones who benefited least were women, and the ones who paid the highest price were children. There is some debate over childhood trauma, such as the breaking of a family and the diagnosis of learning and developmental difficulties or delays. I'm inclined to think there is overlap. High Functioning Autism or Aspergers and Attention Deficit Disorder in girls wasn't a thing in 1980's. You were either with the world and paying attention or you were a daydreamer. I was the latter. I was never formally diagnosed; however, my daughters have since been and so I see in hindsight why I felt my own development so challenging. Whether that is because of genetic predisposition to ASD or ADD or just being sensitive to general environmental arsholery in formative years, I don't know. Maybe it's both. I do know that when I was growing up, I had strong perception of never really fitting in with my peers. Always a few steps behind in comprehension and a strong naivete about how the world really worked created in me a huge vulnerability to predatory personalities. I was the kid who played on my own, who ate on my own, who was needy for friends despite being the target of mean girls. It was easy to befriend girls who would tell me to do things to get me into trouble. If I were a teenager today, I could have easily been convinced I was trans. I'm so thankful for all the struggles because my aspie pattern seeking brain has wrestled with all the why's and done a great deal of learning. The patterns here are very similar and give me slice of hope for my ROGD daughter to come back to herself. As a mother I am compelled to share this hope.

My Great Grandmother was a famous stage actress in England. In many ways she was a product of her time. Most young and beautiful girls go through a narcissistic phase, but once they get to their mid to late 20s will realise the world doesn't revolve around them. From the personal accounts of my great uncle and her son to me directly, her behaviour was described very like a Cluster B, and as my uncle put it, some women should just never be mothers. Of her four children, my grand-father was her golden "Mini-me" child star. He was encouraged into acting at a young age, just as she was. She would dress him up in girl's clothing and adore him with praise that she scarcely had for her other children. I'm not sure that this could be considered normal behaviour by a parent in any context, even though it is happening again today. The process of childhood development is a time of imprinting. My grandfather grew up to develop autogynephilia, alcoholism and had a problem with anger which had a huge effect on his own family life. Sometimes the worst kinds of self-soothing will feed rather than heal the pain we deny, like a drug that can't fill the insatiable hole in the heart. It certainly did break my grandma's heart. My grandparents did not model a healthy relationship to their five children as a direct result of my grandfather's mental, emotional and spiritual state. Sadly, all of their children married very young to leave the dramas of my grandparent's unhappy home behind. They married for all the wrong reasons and had no idea how to relate in healthy ways. All divorced their first spouses. I was the first born and only fruit of one of those marriages which ended after just 18 months. My dad was not a big part of my life for most of my formative years. Growing up I desperately wanted to know my dad personally, just as all little girls do. Every child deserves and developmentally needs both a mother and a father, in a healthy balanced relationship as whole invested parents. It should be a human right, but it's not the world we live in.

My mum married again when I was 8. My new stepdad seemed very likeable and charismatic, funny and kind, but as the years went by, it became apparent that he had a need to be controlling. My new stepsister and stepbrother were much less enthusiastic than I was at the idea of having us as a family. They cast my mum as "the other woman" and have treated her as such to this day. Unfortunately, I became an easy target to take their pain out on. I kept it to myself mostly. Watching my mum get disrespected and seeing her patiently keep on showing kindness to them has been both a blessing and a curse to my heart.

I moved out of home at the age of 21, under the cover of darkness because of the controlling nature of my stepfather, with a boyfriend who I thought I wanted to marry. There was something about him that my mum didn't like, but she couldn't seem to explain to me a good enough reason to not fall in love with him. Even if she did, I wasn't really hearing her. That's how a mother's instinct goes. My beau was five years older than me, newly divorced, had no children, very handsome, tall, charismatic, a bit gregarious, always positive, and best of all, so attentive to want to listen to what I felt and thought about everything. He had a tragic backstory that broke my heart and seemed like a lost puppy. He told me how he was so depressed before he met me and how I was his twin flame, a soul mate for life, that I was the one he had been waiting for and he needed me. I did have an odd feeling that this all seemed a bit over the top, but I decided in my immature pliability that he seemed so confident and genuine. We always had so much fun whenever I was with him it made me want to freeze time and have this kind of relationship always. It's always fun in the beginning. I asked him to marry me after a fit of giggles on one of our car rides, (seeing my ego as a 90s feminist) and he said yes, but it was a long time before we shared that news with anyone. In the meantime, my early years with him were mostly wonderful.

Late one night, early in our relationship, I woke up to use the bathroom and found him watching porn. I was hurt and confused and asked him why he was doing that? He said it was normal for men to watch porn. It made me feel inadequate. We had our first argument about it. He was very forceful to tell me I was being unreasonable and overreacting. I had put aside investing in what few friends I had to be with him and hated the idea of crying to them about something that they might laugh at and felt huge shame around the whole argument, so I buried it and he was sweet again. Little did I know his porn habit would become a major addiction as the years went by, if it wasn't already. I wasn't aware that there was always pressure to compromise my values and the projected shame would erode my personal and emotional boundaries. This is the same for all abusive relationships.

As our wedding date was getting closer, he kept telling me what a wonderful mum I was going to be to our boys and how he was going to teach them to do up Holdens and play rugby. He was insisting that I had to make him a dad before he was 30 because he didn't want to be an old father that couldn't do anything with his kids. Of course, I wanted to please him and agreed to whatever he wanted. We started trying for a baby. I had become accustomed to putting all of his needs and desires first. I felt that his needs and desires were now also mine. I had no concept of what a boundary was, or a clue of what my own likes and preferences were. I revolved around him like the moon to the sun. He could never do any wrong in my eyes. I was totally enmeshed. Our wedding day was magical. We had all our families there and I felt lighter than a feather. We left for our honeymoon the same day, to an island in Malaysia. One of the first things I did after I spotted on our wedding day was to take a pregnancy test which was positive. I thought he would be a lot happier than he seemed at the time.

Morning sickness was unfortunately severe over our honeymoon. One night he wanted to go out to the island nightclub. I agreed for him to go, but I was far too sick to join him. He assured me he would be back by about 10. I was anxious and awake at 3 am when he got back to our room. He laid down next to me and I noticed he completely stopped breathing; I shook him awake and asked what happened to him. He mumbled something about a special drink the band had given him, his words were jumbled and made no sense...

"Did they drug you?" I was already upset.

"Maybe, don't worry I'm fine."

I couldn't sleep then. Looking back, I wonder if it was all a set up to get a reaction out of me, and it worked a treat. I was angry. I wondered how on earth he could act so irresponsibly on our honeymoon. I wondered what I had got myself into and it made me feel so ashamed. I walked around the resort in the early hours of that morning wondering what to do, who to confront, who to complain to. I had a new husband, a baby on the way and no way of knowing if this was a normal experience for a newlywed. Little did I know that day that my experience on what was decidedly a very unhappy honeymoon would be the way our marriage would go every day until I understood exactly the kind of person I was trying to have an unrequited relationship with.

As with our children, there is never a point that they can ever say they are enough and are seen but keep needing to work for a moving line in the sand. The pot of gold at the end of the rainbow is an illusion they have to believe in, or risk excommunication.

The first two years were the best years of our bad marriage. We welcomed our first-born daughter into the world. I was surprised he wasn't too disappointed that she was a girl. He was a great dad to her in her first years of life. Unfortunately, my home visit nurse told me that I couldn't get pregnant when I was breastfeeding. That wasn't good advice. Our second child was born just 18 months later. I decided to find out the gender when I went to have my ultrasound. "You're having a girl" she smiled, and I was flooded with tears of joy. I had always envied my cousin sisters who had each other, did everything together and would forever be best friends. I was so excited to tell my husband that I had quite forgotten he was wanting a boy. His response was not as enthusiastic as mine, but he still seemed happy to me, and asked to name her "Christine"

The night she was born, I was given Nitrous Oxide. It pinned me heavily to the bed for hours so that I couldn't lift my hands or open my eyes. Nobody came to check in on me. My husband was with me, but not saying much as I couldn't communicate. At about 3am a nurse came into my room and told me I was dilated enough. I summoned all my strength and gave one mighty push. I could hear my waters splash on the opposite wall. She was born all at once, but I couldn't open my eyes to see her. I contracted again and my placenta gave way. At that point I had no idea what was happening to me. Everything sounded as if it was down a long tunnel and all I wanted to do was sleep. A woman was saying my name, asking me to stay with her, tapping my hand. It became impossible to tell how many people were in the room as it seemed like 10 hands were massaging my lower abdomen as if it were a big ball of dough. Later I found out that I had had a reaction to the gas and all the capillaries that held my placenta had not closed and I had lost a lot of blood. My husband told me that he had felt sure I was going to die, but oddly he wasn't in the slightest bit upset about any of it. That was something that didn't make much sense to me at the time.

The first year of my daughter's life was difficult. She was colicky, constantly crying and a poor sleeper. Getting up to feed her every time she stirred so as not to disturb my husband's sleep wore me out. It was difficult to get her to sleep without putting her in the car and driving around the block a few times. To make matters worse, our home visit nurse had told us I wasn't allowed to pick her up whenever she cried. I was supposed to let her "cry it out" and let her "self soothe" so that she didn't learn to be manipulative. That was also not the best advice.

Months turned into years and my girls and me, we were happy together. Christine was the sweetest and most loving little angel. Not a bit cheeky, just a genuinely gorgeous hearted kid. I would read to her, sing songs and play games. She loved whatever her big sister loved to do and play with. I made a point of becoming a first educator and invested myself in them both. I brought DK books and flash cards on counting, alphabet and first words. Chistine loved baby dolls, especially a Baby Born doll that she would like to pretend to feed and then sit it on its potty. She loved trying painting, collage crafts, blowing bubbles, soft toys, tea parties, Winnie the Pooh. All the ABC kids shows were favourites, singing along in the car to High 5, reading Spot the Dog lift-the-flap books at bedtime, playdough, pretend baking in a little oven, playing Barbie dress ups… a normal little girl growing up after 2000. Both girls were bright, loving and funny. We had a great bond and relationship.

What changed after Christine's birth was that things at home got more and more lonely. I would have dinner ready, but my husband would say he had to work late, sometimes all night long, to which I naturally appreciated the hard work he was doing for us. We rarely ate together. Sometimes he would come home with lots of money, which he originally led me to believe was his pay. Later I would find out he had a gambling addiction and an apparent allergy to large sums of family inheritance. I didn't understand addiction at all. For most of our marriage we had little money for anything. I had no idea that he had been asking family members for money to cover our family expenses and I was greatly ashamed when I eventually discovered the gravity of his financial irresponsibility. His work circumstances began to shift to a narrative that made my husband a victim of other colleagues within the firm where he was employed. After encouraging him to reach out to contacts to find another job, we moved far away from my family to a rural area for a simpler lifestyle. I thought it would give him more time to spend with us. Instead, he decided he needed time to go fishing with locals in order to establish himself in the small community. I could see Christine was suffering as she longed for her daddy to come home to spend time with us all. It triggered my own memory of wanting my own dad and it pressed me into asking my husband to stay home with us and invest his time and attention in our daughters. He always had an excuse to promise just a few months more and everything would be perfect again. Years passed and nothing really changed. I focused on getting our daughters into a routine with some stability. Locals seemed to think my husband was a bit of a celebrity. He changed his personality and became just like them in every way. I was starving for the old him, the person that he was toward me when we first met. I sometimes couldn't tell if he was being a diplomat or a fraud, but I wanted to give him the benefit of the doubt.

The Karpman Drama Triangle is a pattern of behaviour where we see someone believing they are a victim and projecting their own failures onto someone else as a perpetrator. It can also be called splitting/ good object/ bad object. Common in personality disordered thinking and mental illness. They are usually unaware that they are enjoying casting themselves as a martyr or hero to the wider community, while simultaneously calling themselves oppressed as a victim. They usually also have a part of themselves that feels justified in a narrative that gives them permission to rage at whomever they perceive as their oppressor, and in fact are a villain themselves, feigning hurt that the response they have received somehow proves their point. And so, the drama continues of their own creating, apparently oblivious to their own hand in it all. The Karpman Drama

Triangle is not new, rather a pattern common to humanity through all of time. My first husband definitely lived in a Karpman drama triangle.

I became so desperate for change, that I asked my husband if he would like to try to have the baby boy he had always wanted. Would a son make him want to spend more time with us as a family? It's this day my mind keeps going back to. Why did I say such a thing? Why did I make myself so vulnerable? He knew my weaknesses. He knew my family history and knew why I didn't have a dad growing up. His reply came so quickly, like he'd rehearsed it a hundred times to know exactly where to twist the knife. In the hearing of Christine, who was only about 6 at the time, he quickly answered, "Christine is my boy". At this he lavished her with his attention, affection and praise. She lit up like a Christmas tree. After that, Christine decided she didn't want to wear anything pink or any of her previously loved dresses anymore, but never did she ask for actual boy's clothes. I told my husband as well as his family, that I thought it was wrong of him to call her that. As usual, I was told that I was the one being silly. She played in to his fantasy game and asked me to buy her cars and Tonka trucks. They got put in a drawer, and slid under her bed, untouched and in perfect condition for years. What she wanted was her dad's investment in her. Away from extended family, I was the only one who was seeing any of it firsthand. It broke my heart to see him shower her with crumbs of affection for five minutes and then disappear to drink beer with some bloke we hardly knew down the road for the rest of the evening, expecting Christine and the rest of us to believe we'd just had weeks of high-quality time.

Finally, the day came when my husband brought home another "friend". A woman this time, 15 years his junior. They became very close which was hard for the girls and I to watch. She lavished us all with gifts and tried to be my friend. I wanted to believe her. I tried to be what my husband was asking me to be. When the girls weren't around, I would go to them both privately and tell them how their "friendship" was hurting the girls as well as our marriage and could they please respect my boundaries and not invest themselves so heavily in each other. Yet again, I was being the unreasonable one – jealous, possessive, and full of self-inflicted imagination. They were above reproach and how dare I tarnish their good reputations in the community with my outlandish accusations! His friend was trying so hard to be there for me and babysit our girls so that he could have the opportunity to spend more time with me... just as soon as he had some money to go out with, which never came. They were so relentless in their gaslighting that I really did start to think maybe I was the one with the problem, that maybe I was going crazy. I would apologise in humiliation on multiple occasions. Then the slander behind my back began. They were, of course, having a full-blown affair and keeping me completely in the dark by telling me that everything I was seeing was all in my head and I needed my husband to tell me what was real and what wasn't. To make matters worse, he quit his job and refused to look for another one, money was scarce, we had to go to Vinnies for food and financial help. I wasn't sleeping, lost a lot of weight and developed several health problems.

I decided to see our family GP. By this stage I had come to live in fear, trying to hold myself and our family together with wishes and prayers. After pouring out my heart to our doctor, telling him I was terrified I was losing my hold on reality, he said to me "I've seen your hubby around town, and I'd like you to tell him I'm a bit concerned about him and could he please make an appointment to come see me". I felt like I was conspiring something, that I would be found out and I would be laughed at and ridiculed. I was trying hard to not allow my mental health to decline further so I found the courage and passed on the message as if it was from a phone call. About 6 weeks later my doctor called me back into his office. "Your husband says he knows exactly what he's doing to you, and he knows it's not right, but he doesn't care. He actually had the audacity to tell me he is enjoying it and has no intention of changing. The only way to help your marriage is you must leave him".

This day was my absolute rock bottom.

I was gobsmacked and sat completely dumbfounded at what my family doctor had just disclosed. A minute later however, I felt a surge of anger, but not at my husband, at the doctor!

"How can you tell me to destroy my own family?"

I was accusing myself of what my husband was doing, just as he would accuse me of doing all of the things he was doing behind my back. I had become "infected" with similar thought patterns through abuse. Accusations are confessions.

Thankfully I had sense enough to take my doctor's next advice, which was to see a therapist. She heard my story and referred me to Al-Anon Family groups, which at first, I resisted. After all, wasn't she telling me that it wasn't my fault? At Al-Anon I learnt about my own codependent, people pleasing behaviour. I learnt what a boundary was and how to assert one respectfully. To know a boundary may cost me something but is ultimately acting for my own highest good. I learnt what detachment was and started valuing detachment as a virtue. There was so much love and support at those meetings. I soon saw the toxic dance I was contributing to and began to recognise and change my previous fawning behaviours and emotional, black and white thinking. I got a sponsor who I could call any time and found sanity in her wisdom. I worked on that program like my life depended on it. Believing if I gave it my all, then I might win back my husband as he was in the beginning, but that was magical thinking. Little did I realise the problem was much bigger than addiction. Many hours at the library reading through book after book to try to figure out where on earth I was at with myself, how I got there and what I could do to get better was very limited. It wasn't until finally recognising the pattern in the 12-step program is a spiritual awakening and working the program deeply that I began to search for a personal relationship with God. Often abusers hate spirituality and will quickly show the truth of who they really are at the sight or sound of prayer. Religiosity is also the perfect place for abusers to hide. The facade of perfection is shallow, and people rely on others never looking too deeply into a matter so as to appear rude or embarrassed to be seen meddling in the affairs of what is proclaimed to be virtuous. So too there is a gnostic religiosity to the trans belief.

When Christine turned 8 years old, my first husband left me to be with his lady friend. He didn't make it obvious, by moving in with his parents first. No doubt to tell them what a hopeless excuse for a wife I was. The absence of emotional tension in the home refreshed me with space to breath, relax and start to focus on the girls' needs. When I would ask my oldest how she was feeling, she was able to articulate at the tender age of 9 that she didn't like how her dad treated me but, given she was concerned that if she told him that, he might treat her the same way as he was treating me. She felt helpless to do anything and became angry towards men. Nobody wants that for their daughter. There are still good men in the world, and she deserved to know that. When I asked Christine how she was doing, she would always respond the same thing in a baby voice, "I'm a puppy, no, I'm going to be a bunny rabbit! Hop, hop, hop!" She was disassociating. Possibly even not knowing what emotion she was feeling at all. Somebody once said, "reinvention is an excellent form of avoidance" and I have to agree. I wonder if my daughter as well as many of our children are using the same avoidance and dissociative coping strategy in a futile attempt to erase past hurts.

I took both girls to see the Community Services Family Councillor. I'm not sure it was much help. Christine's grades at school got worse. Her teacher told me she was regressing academically, and I saw the same at home. She was wetting her bed at night, wanting to sleep with the lights on or with me. My instincts as a mother told me she didn't want to face the pain of divorce we were all feeling, and that she was hiding in a denial that was protecting her. I knew in my gut that her bottled up feelings of rejection and unmet needs from him would eventually come out in ugly ways that I just could never predict. I hate that I was right. I just tried to show her love and encourage her to express her feelings which she always struggled to articulate, and spent as much time with her as I could. I have never felt that all my love or all the family counselling was enough to make up for those unmet needs.

About four months after their dad left, I finally found a casual job cleaning at a local nursing home. My shifts began at 6am and ended at 6pm. With no family support around me, I paid a neighbour to wake them up in the morning and get them ready for school. Christine was very un-co-operative and never wanted to get out of bed in the morning. Our neighbour was what polite people might call a rough diamond. She had a mouth like a sailor. Not used to taking orders from someone she considered verbally abusive, Christine decided to hide under the house and our neighbour couldn't find her. My helper quit that day. Our eldest had to try to get Christine to school and on the bus instead. In later years our eldest daughter told me that she felt like she had to be the parent, which she should never have been burdened with. I knew I couldn't stay where I was and be the mum they needed me to be at the same time. They needed their dad to come back and love us. So after I had been working at the nursing home for about 3 months and I felt stable, I decided to write a letter to my husband because he never ever answered my phone calls or texts. I needed to tell him about how Christine was regressing and how I wanted our marriage back as it was in the beginning. We all needed the old him back, but stressed if he wanted a divorce, he needed to tell me. About 2 months later he phoned as if about something unrelated to my letter.

"Did you get my letter?" I pressed for his answer.

Then came the barrage,

"Yes, I do want a divorce, because we are just too different, but you absolutely needed to know that I have always been a very faithful husband to you. There won't be anyone else for me, I'm never getting married again and I'm not seeing that other woman (he married her actually). I'm not going to be able to pay any child support for a while because I have to pay off all of our debts from family loans when I didn't have a job for over a year and you had better be thankful for living rent free in our half-finished house".... on and on the "dramatic victim" narrative went...

I was numb and didn't know how to move forward. I leaned hard into prayer and my 12 steps that gave me clarity and stability. I grieved the loss of what I had hoped would return to me as it once was, but it was all only an illusion I wanted to see. Reality broke my denial and physically my body went into actual shock. I cried all the time, had panic attacks whenever I saw a car like his lady friend's, had nightmares, memory fog, ruminating over and over. Unusually, had a hard time remembering day to day arrangements and felt like a failure as a parent. I was angry at myself too — how could I have been so stupid to give my daughters such a father?

My family told me to put our half-built home on the market. Offers were made but he never accepted any of them. I went to see someone from Legal Aid and lodged divorce papers for shared custody to begin legal proceedings. I continued at Al Anon for support through my grief on my shifts off work and tried as always to get more intentional about bringing stability to our daughters. With the help of extended family and newfound friends, I did manage to create some happy memories with our girls amid a painful year.

One day when I was collecting a single parent subsidy from Centrelink, there was a small flyer on the pinboard dividers between the desks. It was offering ex government refurbished computers with internet connections for anyone on a single parent benefit. I ordered one on the spot. When the computer finally arrived, I set it up and registered myself on Facebook and tried to think of all the people I had known when I was young, focusing on family friends who I believed had integrity and I could trust. One of those people was a family friend who I had met as a teenager in England. His Stepmum and my Mum had been best friends since school. He had separated from his first wife and was living in New Zealand. I remembered he was sweet on me when we were kids for the brief holiday visit we had. His profile showed me he had become a skydiving instructor and a motorbike enthusiast, into Bear Grylls style survival skills, tramping and rock climbing. Nothing like me at all. Clicking the friend request button, I wondered if he would remember me. Within hours he had accepted, and we messaged back and forth, catching up on the past 20 years. He heard my story and had a lot of insight and practical wisdom for me as his own stepfather had treated his mum in a similar way. I was comforted by his understanding. After about 6 months of chatting, he came out to Sydney to meet us all. We walked around the harbour and it felt like we had picked up where we left off. I was very wary, but his investment in my life was like food to someone starving. When I saw him off at the airport, he kissed me goodbye and said "I'm coming back for you". For the first time in a long time, I felt seen and loved. Being the mum I wanted to be on my own had proved to be impossible for me. I desperately wanted the chance to share life with someone who wanted to share life with me and build a healthy family life together. Many single parents do a wonderful job on their own. People don't always appreciate how hard it is to do that well.

Early the following year, I was invited to New Zealand to meet my new boyfriend's family. He asked me to marry him. I accepted and went home to tell my daughters that I was going to be able to be a full-time mum to them again, that they would have a new Stepdad and we would be moving to New Zealand to be with him. In telling my ex-husband about my engagement, he said he was extremely happy for me and explained to me that if my new husband wanted to adopt the girls as his own, he had his blessing. This grandiosity felt very strange to me, like a psychological and emotional trap. His reaction to me leaving the country with our children was so over the top it left me wondering what on earth he was thinking. How was he ok to just let our daughters go out of his life and into my full custody completely? Had he ever really wanted them at all? Would he change his mind and get customs to stop us at the airport? Whatever the reason, I instinctively felt he was playing mind games with me, and my heart was in my mouth the entire flight to New Zealand. I didn't rest until we were in our new home. In hindsight I think it was child support accountability that he didn't want. Our daughters were uneasy about everything which was totally understandable, but they were happy at the promise of getting me back and that's what I thought was a step in the right direction. Christine adored my new fiancé. She even started to take his surname when she wrote her name on things.

We enrolled the girls in a small country school outside of the town we lived in. They arrived emotionally and mentally traumatised and in deep need of attention without having the words or awareness to understand how they were seen by others. The teachers were filled with so much compassion for us, nurtured the girls' obvious emotional wounds and Christine's learning difficulties. We were told she had dyslexia, ADD, anxiety and some other processing and learning difficulties. Very recently a therapist has told her she has High Functioning Autism.

My feeling is that it could just be that she had come from a very unsettling environment but what do I know. The efforts of the teachers bred in them success and they began some surface healing. Christine became head girl in her final year of middle school. They both began to blossom into the young women I was hoping to raise them as. Christine grew her hair long down her back and even wore dresses occasionally. She had no idea how pretty she was. Watching her look up to her big sister and see their bond really develop was balm to my soul. They would spend girly time together with manicures and makeup, creative time, giggly bonding time, sleepovers with mutual friends and days out to various family activities. My new husband would take them out for ice-cream after dinner. He is also a pilot, so not only skydiving but flying in a two-seater and extreme fun at Adventure parks were some of the family times we shared with the girls. We sent them on youth camping trips and made sure they had plenty of time with their new friends. I was mindful not to lug them with too many chores or minding the two new baby siblings we added to our family, too much. I really wanted them to have a good life with all the extra-curricular activities and tuition they liked.

About a year after we had settled into our new life in New Zealand, Christine decided she would like to learn Karate. We made a booking for an after-school class. At first, she practised the kata without any problem. The sparring was not so easy. One afternoon when my new husband picked her up, he arrived early to watch her spar. She was getting pummelled and hurt. It was clear she was trying to keep a stiff upper lip. My new husband has a soft spot for Christine, he reassured her that she didn't have to do this if she didn't want to. After some thought she told him "I suppose I don't need to protect Mum anymore". We were surprised at this small insight into her thinking. She earned her yellow belt and didn't go back again.

When our eldest daughter finished high school, she decided to move to another city to study Speech Pathology at university. We thought that her moving away might affect Christine in a negative way, so we sold our home to move to the same city to be close to her. Both girls had been attending an all-girls high school and did very well there. Christine was happy, getting good grades and had nice friends. In hindsight I wish we had stayed where we were until she also had finished high school. I had no reason to believe the next school she attended wouldn't have her best interest at heart.

We moved in April 2017. The road trip was fun, with snacks and car karaoke. We arrived at our new home in the Easter school holidays and had a week to gather new uniforms and enrol in new schools. The school uniforms in New Zealand for girls are ankle length kilts. Some sort of Kiwi tradition from Scotland I'm guessing. Christine did not want to wear the massive unflattering skirt. "Think of it as a blanket," I suggested. She wasn't impressed. For the first two weeks she seemed happy enough when she got home from school. We made an appointment to see the school Dean for her year to check that she was making good friends, settling into classes ok and were assured that she had made friends with some quality students who would encourage her to keep her good grades and keep up her previously enjoyed success. We had also previously organised an academic evaluation for a reader writer for her final exams, which we had wanted the staff at the new school to be familiar with so that Christine had the best chance with her finals. About four weeks after she started, I got a phone call from the school counsellor to say, "Christine really didn't want me to call you because she loves you so much, but we have to tell you she is suicidal, and could you please take her to your family GP today?"

This was just unbelievable.

When Christine got home, we asked her what was going on and she brushed it off like it was silly. She assured us she was fine and in absolutely no danger. I asked why I needed to take her to the GP? She just said it was something she had told the school counsellor in confidence from years past and she was totally fine. We took her to the GP anyway. Only having registered with them a few days earlier nobody knew us at all. We were asked to stay out of the room while Christine had her consultation. That was also a first. The door eventually opened, and I asked the Doctor, "Is she? Do we need to be worried?" The Doctor assured me that my daughter was definitely not suicidal, and there was nothing to worry about. It was a relief but also left us wondering what on earth was going on. Christine had usually been honest in our relationship with her so we gave her the benefit of the doubt and decided to trust her. That was the first mistake on day one of the nightmare that was about to unfold.

Christine's new friends seemed very different from her old friends. They had the liberty of no dress code at school for hair colours and piercings and while we thought it was not what we would prefer to see her emulate, we know differentiation is a stage all teenagers go through. It gradually became apparent that they all self-identified as somewhere on the LGBT rainbow. We thought, as long as they were applying themselves to their schooling, what did it matter?

But it did matter.

As the weeks turned into months, Christine's grades and personality began to decline badly. Depression and moodiness were new battles for us as a family; she was spending more and more time as a recluse in her room. It was hard to get her to go to bed, hard to get her out of bed in the morning, hard to get her off the internet, which she claimed was for homework. Hard to get her off her phone, hard to get her to pack lunch during the day and most of all hard to get her to really be open and talk to us honestly like she once did. All of this can seem somewhat normal for a lot of teenagers, so I tried to be lenient with her, but my mother's intuition told me something was off. I started to ask her if something was wrong but she would change the subject. I asked her if her new friends were experimenting with drugs or alcohol, is that why she was acting oddly? "No Mum, I'm not taking drugs, don't be stupid!" Did she also identify as her new friends did, as a lesbian? Negative again. I asked her if she was struggling with sexuality? She said she thought she might be Bi, but she really didn't like the idea of sex at all. After listing a whole lot of possibilities that might be making her act so out of character, I finally wormed out of her that she thought she might be Trans. After all of the other things that I had thought of that seemed far worse, I initially felt, "Oh is that all?" At that time, I thought it just meant cross dressing and wasn't bothered in the slightest. A few weeks later she asked me what her name would have been if she had been born a boy and I told her. This is the new name she used behind our back at school. We would sometimes hear her new friends call her that boy's name and I asked her about it. "It's just a nickname" she insisted "We play D and D and make up names for each-other all the time" One of her other new friends also had changed her name a few times, so we bought her lie. She asked me if she could go to an Armageddon Convention dressed in Cosplay for her 17th birthday. I had a background in costumes and fashion design, so I agreed. We went to Spotlight for craft materials to create a Jack Frost costume. Part of the costume she asked for was a binder, which I agreed to for the costume. The weeks passed and the supplies sat in the wardrobe, but the binder went on and barely ever came off. This was the big clue that she wasn't being honest with us. She had seen her dad continually gaslight me and now I had the same feelings from her. It broke my heart. At that point I decided it was time to do some research into what being "Trans" actually meant these days. This led me to papers by Dr Paul McHugh from the 1970s. It was horrifying to learn the full extent of his research. John Hopkins Hospital had closed sex change surgeries because patients would become 40 times more likely at risk of suicide 7 to 10 years after transition compared to those who did not. This was also confirmed in a Swedish study. So why was it being pushed onto the most vulnerable and impressionable? Back in 2017, research on the long-term effects on testosterone in a woman's body was hard to find for a tech newbie like me. It made sense that as hormones are made of cholesterol, that massive amounts would have the ability to line the arteries and lead to atherosclerosis, which is the leading cause of heart disease. I decided to look at the reason why kids thought they were the opposite sex and watched video diary after video diary of transitioning teens on YouTube. They all said the same thing like auditioning for a part in a play! All were hugely self-absorbed, checking themselves out in their video mirrors and speaking for 10 minutes without saying very much at all. It was nothing like the Christine we knew. Listening to a panel of "professionals" presenting explanations of all things transgender, I initially heard that everything was totally reversible. This since has been proven misinformation but has not yet been removed from mainstream belief. Censorship only goes one way apparently. The woman was spouting that if you decide you want boobs again you can just go get some! How do you breast feed a baby with fake boobs? The more I discovered, the more distressed I became. I asked Christine if I could come to one of her therapy sessions, thinking I could listen to some of the deeper issues in her heart to get some insight into why she felt this way. Perhaps the therapist would also benefit from learning some of my perspective.

She agreed for me to come to the last of the six sessions with the therapist she was seeing through school at our local GP's office. I was again told to wait outside, and they would call me in when they were ready. My hopes that I would at least be able to contribute some of her family backstory were disappearing as time kept ticking away. Finally with 10 minutes left on the hour session I was called in. The first thing I noticed was Christine shaking all over and white as a sheet like she was in some sort of shock and wouldn't look at me in my eyes. The therapist told me that if Christine didn't transition that she would suicide, and it was better for me to have a live son than a dead daughter. From that day forward we all needed to call him by his chosen name and never use his "dead" birth name again. We were to expect him to begin taking testosterone and soon expect surgery for a double mastectomy through ACC, Accident Compensation Commission, New Zealand's Government funded healthcare. In careful desperation I turned in earnest and tried to talk to my baby girl, "Honey, we love you the way you are, you don't have to do this, we don't care how you dress or what haircut you have, we love you just as you are. Can I ask exactly why you don't want to be Christine anymore?" No reply ever came, she was hunched over in a chair turned away from me as if I was a monster. Turning my conversation to the therapist I asked, "Are you not interested in my understanding of my daughter and how there are very likely valid psychological reasons why she might feel the way she does? Do you not need to understand her past?" The therapist policed my pronouns and spoke over the top of me, while she busied herself at her computer. Not the slightest bit interested in looking at me in the eye, speaking with me or hearing anything from my perspective. I found it very hard to believe this woman had any empathy in her at all as it was clear I was being emotionally blackmailed and cut off. I felt abused again. It was very clear that anything I had to say would not make any difference. This was the extent of my input to her therapy, a brick wall. I was beyond hurt. I was angry.

Driving Christine back to school that day I desperately tried to reason with her heart. "Honey, I feel like you're trying to somehow kill off my daughter, and I love her, I have always loved her and I always will. I cannot allow you to take testosterone under my roof when your little sister and brother, who idolise you and want to copy everything you do, are watching what happens to you. This will break the heart of everyone who loves you. You don't need to do this to yourself. Why on earth do you not want to hear me?" Telling her about the medical dangers that were likely but largely unknown barely raised an eyebrow. None of my concerns were felt a good enough reason to not medicalise. She was invincible. Nothing bad was ever going to happen to her under the care of medical professionals, and even if I could explain it, I'm not sure she would have heard me. Now I understood how my own Mother felt. The more I warned with tears the more she disengaged, and the emotional distance grew wider as if I was insane. All she could say to me was "I've always felt this way, I don't see what the big deal is". Telling me she had always felt male was a huge red flag. I would have seen it when she was growing up, because of her dad calling her "his boy". In meeting other parents, it became obvious that she was actually just following a script that I hadn't seen at the time. I did however, recognise the spirit of the behaviour as the same spirit of the battle in my first marriage which is why I refused to play that game again.

Learning everything I could became an all-encompassing obsession. I tried to find her a therapist who would address her childhood dissociative trauma and not affirm her delusions, but it was 2018 and after my experience I had little trust for any doctor or therapist. In my desperation I enrolled myself in a college to become a family therapist myself. I think I must have indicated a strong desire for objective truth as grounding for mental health in my first paper, because the Head of the College came to me privately and said they would only be teaching narrative therapy, a postmodern therapy that only allowed for a client to tell their own story as they believed it to be their own version of the truth.

"What about the fact that people lie to themselves all the time? Aren't we supposed to help them think critically?"

"No, we don't tell them anything" I was told "Have you considered becoming a Life Coach?"

I left the college with at least some understanding of what healthy human development looks like.

Someone I admire once said, "If a person says they care about mental health yet have no interest in prioritising reason and critical thinking skills, they don't understand what being mentally healthy is, nor do they understand the purpose of therapy". It's no wonder we are now hearing de-transitioners telling us that being in "therapy" only made them worse. Therapists have damaged their own reputations by agreeing to buy into what they should have known was not ethical from the beginning. They have lied to themselves and as a result have lost all credibility. It's no wonder people are hungry for Jordan Peterson content. As he has said, "There are falsehoods so deep that they are the exact opposite of the truth. Sexually reproducing creatures, even without nervous systems can tell the difference between male and female. If you can get people to swallow the lie that there is no difference between men and women, then there is no lie they won't swallow".

One morning in late 2018, I was awake at 3am as I had been for many nights before. The only relief I found from my anxiety and tears was in scripture, fasting and deep long hours of prayer. As I had been learning to lean into my faith, I felt a very clear still voice speak to my heart.

"You have to let her go and live with her dad".

"No! God Please! Anything but that!"

"You have to let her go and live with her dad".

Something deep within me knew it was true. I cried softly. I didn't want to let her go.

"Trust me".

"I do trust You God, I can't do any of this without You strengthening me".

Three days passed and all I could think about was having to let her go. On the third morning Christine came to me and said "Mum, I've been thinking I'd like to move back to Australia to spend some time with my dad for a while".

"Yes," I said quietly, and I gave her a hug. "It's ok, you can go".

She seemed a bit shocked but surprised in a good way, hugged me and thanked me. Then skipped away to organise her big move back to Australia, to no doubt be affirmed as a boy by her dad again. After her exams that year, all of which she failed, except for photography, she was packed and on a plane for the Christmas holidays. We tried to stay in contact together for most of 2019 after she left. I was always careful not to call her a pronoun at all, but my term of endearment name I have called her all her life to know my love has never changed for her.

I got a phone call from Christine in early 2020, just before lockdown, telling me she was about to begin taking testosterone. I was totally devastated. I begged her not to do it. We were both crying, but she told me she just had to do this, as if she didn't have a choice and wouldn't tell me why. It didn't make sense at the time, but it makes me wonder if she was ever really in the driver's seat of that decision. Soon I saw her Facebook page had changed to male and all the love bombing she was getting online from my own family members. I went into a deep depressive grief, an anguish I had never experienced even at the hand of her father. Everyone I thought had her best interest at heart had completely disregarded my heart for my girl. Physical, emotional, mental and spiritual torturous pain that never seemed to end. It frightened me to the point of wondering if I might need to be sedated in a hospital. My new husband watched helplessly and cried with me, not knowing how to comfort me. The physical chest pain I experienced frightened me too. Insomnia, difficulty being present in my life, crying all the time, distrust for everyone who I thought loved my family all returned like bad DeJa'Vu . Once again, I had to work out where on earth I was. Day by day I made a deliberate choice to put myself back together again for my new husband and small children who deserved the best of me. This time it wasn't my own people pleasing and fawning behaviour that got me in pain. It was strangers and people I thought were friends and my own family. The depth of anger at the audacity to take my daughter away from me thinking they are doing a great virtuous moral service stirred so much anger in me I barely recognised myself. It still seems too much to forgive and impossible to restore. Who do they think they are to define good and evil for themselves? I saw the reality of who others are as I used to be, and I was utterly disgusted with humanity at how easily we are all so manipulated by lies, group think and full on unfounded fear. This is a shadow we need to look at for a long time.

During lockdown in 2020 Christine refused to respond to any of my messages as I kept trying to show her love. I had been fasting and praying more and more to cope and as I began to heal, I felt a clear knowing in my heart she would soon move to a popular seaside town close to my parent's house and she would then work things out on her own and realise she can never be a man, without anyone else's influence. My mum phoned me in February 2021 to tell me that Christine had been in a bad way, that she was no longer living with her dad, but had been homeless and living in someone's garage throughout 2020. Suddenly, I understood why she hadn't wanted to talk to me and wondered if starting testosterone and lockdown had made her somehow unable to continue living with her dad. She became deeply in debt and seemingly couldn't manage money. My parents bailed her out and expected us to pay them back. Respectfully we told them Christine would never learn responsibility if she got bailed out all the time. She needed to have a payment plan in place once she had a job to re-pay her debts herself. We had given her the "The Barefoot Investor" book by Scott Pape years before, and she had read it and had started to work on his program as soon as she had left our care a year earlier. There really was no excuse. Mum then told me Christine was going to be moving in with them for a while until she found a place in the same coastal town that God had whispered to my heart months before. I was flooded with peace and hope. By faith I believe God has Christine in His hands, by evidence of things coming to pass and yet to happen. He's bigger than all of it, for all of our children.

Many parents struggle with the idea of forgiveness because the pain is so intense and prolonged, They suffer physically, emotionally and spiritually. I'd like to offer that you forgive in your own time. Don't be shamed or bullied into having to forgive in order to be a "good parent". Forgiveness is not a feeling or a licence to say hurt is permissible. It is a practice of spiritual warfare and a choice of the Will that is present progressive. Forgiveness has very little to do with feelings. The biggest hurdle is to try to identify with the humanity of someone who behaves as a Cluster B personality. These personality types have a way of being charming when they want to be, but for all the wrong reasons. This is the hard part to identify with and why we struggle. There is no way any of what has been lost can ever be restored. Forgiveness at its heart is knowing the Gospel, that we are all "born that way" to some degree. Making a decision to pick up our own cross to follow Jesus because of what God has forgiven us, is our own personal choice. There is never any coercion in the one true God.

My childhood family have believed Christine and her dad's narrative that I am the problem. That I have been an irresponsible parent and not had her best interests at heart. My refusal to face "facts" that "she" is a "he" is solely what is making her so depressed and as such I am no longer worthy to be a part of the family or her life. My stepdad has told every person in his extended family that I'm no longer welcome at any of the extended family gatherings, and as far as I am aware they have obeyed him as there have been no more invites to any gatherings. Personally, I think it's good to know who your friends are. Today Christine has continued to alienate herself from me completely, despite me reaching out to her with gifts on her birthdays and messages of love. Parental alienation says much more about the one doing the alienating than the one being alienated.

When a parent loses a child, or has a self-harming child, part of their own healing is to advocate against what has hurt them, in the loving memory of who they knew their child to be. As part of my own healing process, I have become involved in raising awareness of what governments, teachers and medical professionals are doing to create ROGD kids in schools and usurping parental authority. I participate in various online support groups, staying connected and encouraging other parents at various stages of the same trauma. I am also working through a political outlet to campaign via a Citizens Initiated Referendum to get gender ideology out of New Zealand classrooms.

My hope for our beloved Christine is that she comes to understand that everybody has a hole in their heart where a loving parent should be. She might consider that missing parent as me, but I am a poor substitute to truly fill that hole. I'm not God. Nobody can parent like Him. I hope she comes to know a personal relationship with Jesus. My prayer is that someday soon a light goes on in her mind and she will awake to see she can never be a man, swallow her pride and stop living in futility. I want her to know she only has one body in this life and if she doesn't respect it, where will she live? Life is about way more than mere sexuality or gender, but it's not right to harm those things in people. I hope that there is a way to restore her health in a natural and gentle way.

I want every family to know there is no such thing as being born in the wrong body, and that nobody can change their sex. Queer theory is designed at its core to erase families in a thousand different ways. It steals our kid's history, their critical thinking, their affections and their very future. Since the Cass Review and the WPATH files have been released, there are no more excuses. Their fraudulence and malpractice have been exposed. It's now just a matter of time before justice is completely served. I will advocate this cause for the rest of my life, and I know other parents all over the world stand with me. I hope that my story will contribute to how therapists see the damage that has been done to families and the generational trauma for women and children of fatherlessness. There will be many women who have been through testosterone whom in my opinion, deserve free health care to undo the damage of what testosterone has done to their bodies and minds as they begin to understand the self-harm and bad advice that was inflicted. It is precisely the ADD, the ADHD and ASD traits that will eventually drive them to dig much deeper into understanding the why of things and this will undo their current beliefs. Our children will not be able to live in denial once the layers of lies fall off over time. We have to be there for them in these high-risk years.

Looking forward, it's only a matter of time before this toxic rainbow disappears, and our children understand how they were hoodwinked guinea pigs in a political and medical scandal that has left them sterile with sexual dysfunction. I can only imagine how devastating that will be to come to terms with. They will need our support. If we can show them how to navigate through their journey of healing, I believe they are destined to become some of the most spiritual, wise and beautiful people the world will ever have the pleasure knowing. No parent could be more blessed than to stand beside our de transitioned children, help them regain their health, and fight the good fight alongside them for justice in one of the greatest medical crimes in living memory.

Lawsuits are coming.

Thank you for hearing me.

CHAPTER 10

How did the media get it so wrong?

After several years of censoring negative stories about children's gender treatments, it is encouraging to note that the tide appears to be turning. The mainstream media has in the past few years demonstrated a renewed willingness to report on this issue. As some practitioners working in the field and young de-transitioners break ranks and speak out publicly, media coverage has followed suit, albeit reluctantly, in reporting significant developments to date.

The debate surrounding children and young people undergoing gender treatments and surgery has been unnecessarily shrouded in secrecy, with any dissent or counter-narrative to the wholehearted affirmation of gender treatments for children or young people actively being ignored or censored by the media. Given the experimental nature of these treatments, a media environment that refuses to report transparently on this issue puts children and young people at risk of grave harm, and does a disservice to desperate parents wanting to access information that helps them to care for their children in the best way they can.

As outlined by the Australian newspaper in an editorial[1] following the closure of the Tavistock clinic in England:

> Parents and children in need deserve to know the treatments they are being offered do not fall outside mainstream mental health guidelines or have been motivated by hardcore transgender ideology.

Given that gender treatments are experimental and that few, if any, have been subject to long term studies or experiments[2], the risks to children and young people are high. Relying on the child to be the 'expert' in their life and about their gender and identity is a risky approach. A media that refuses to report on these issues is complicit in harming children.

The issue was barely on the public's radar ten years ago. And yet, during this period, the numbers of children and young people presenting to gender clinics 'exploded' with "gender services in Australia, as well as throughout the West ... struggling to keep pace with surging demand"[3].

The dramatic increase in the numbers of children and young people being referred for gender treatment has made it far more difficult for the issue to be ignored by the media. The fact of some young people ceasing their transition treatments, and speaking out, as well as other practitioners also speaking up, has meant that the issue could no longer be ignored, despite the pressure brought by pro-affirmation treatment activists.

An important development which has resulted in the significant increase in children receiving these treatments was the removal of the need for judicial oversight for each phase of hormonal treatment (which was the case previously). As reported[4] in the Australian newspaper:

> Persuaded by gender clinicians and human rights lawyers, the Family Court had made it easier over the past several years for children and adolescents to get puberty-blocker drugs, cross-sex hormones and surgery such as mastectomy without the obstacle of a court application, as long as parents did not disagree.

---

1 Editorial, "Gender treatments need review', *The Australian*, 30 July 2022.

2 Dr Hilary Cass, *Independent Review of gender identity services for children and young people: Final Report, April 2024*: https://cass.independent-review.uk/home/publications/final-report/

3 Julie Szego, "A question of transition gender treatment under scrutiny" 4 June 2023, Substack, accessed here https://szegounplugged.substack.com/p/a-question-of-transition

4 Editorial, "Gender treatments need review', *The Australian*, 30 July 2022.

As an editorial[5] in the Australian newspaper noted, "the sharp growth in claims of gender dysphoria, particularly by young women who feel they should be male, is a confronting trend that requires serious attention."

In December 2020, the Australian[6] reported on the British High Court ruling against the NHS Tavistock youth gender clinic on medical treatments for transgender and non-binary children.

This was a pivotal moment in the discourse regarding gender treatment for children and young people. The British High Court's ruling against the NHS Tavistock youth gender clinic in December 2020 challenged the prevailing assertion that puberty blockers are a lifesaving, fully reversible and harmless intervention for transgender and non-binary children. The case, brought by Keira Bell, a 23-year-old who regretted her transition which she began at 16, underscored the irreversible and profound implications of such medical treatments. Kiera Bell's testimony highlighted the stark realities of fertility and identity loss, directly challenging the narrative that these treatments are without significant risk.

This is a highly significant decision that has profoundly affected the treatment of children and young people in the UK who are experiencing gender dysphoria.

Media outlets have proved themselves to be either reluctant or unwilling to report on these issues generally, a fact which Julie Szego, a journalist working at the Age newspaper for twenty years, discovered recently. In her own words, she was met with blockage after blockage when trying to report on stories about de-transitioners or women's protests such as the Let Women Speak protest in Melbourne.

And while Newscorp newspapers the Australian, Daily Telegraph and Herald Sun initially reported on these issues, the Australian newspaper's coverage of trans issues (in particular) came under fire after Dr Michelle Telfer, previous director of the gender clinic at the Royal Children's Hospital in Melbourne made a complaint to the Australian Press Council for its reporting[7]:

---

5 Ibid.

6 Bernard Lane, "Kiera Bell, gender transition and the lifelong damage of a puberty blue", *The Australian*, 5 December 2020.

7 Zoe Samios, "'Substantial distress': Press Watchdog rebukes The Australian for reporting on gender issues", *Sydney Morning Herald*, 3 September 2021.

The Australian's articles were published between August 9, 2019 and June 29, 2020. They discussed transgender children and teenagers, the safety and ethics of giving hormone treatment to young people experiencing gender dysphoria and the rates of de-transitioning in transgender young people. Almost all the pieces were written by Bernard Lane, The Australian's roving editor, data journalist and leader writer. One article was written by Jennifer Oriel and the remaining articles in question were editorials.

The Press Council found that the Australian's reporting on this issue was in the public interest, but partially upheld a complaint by Dr Telfer.

Julie Szego was subsequently[8] sacked from her position at the Age newspaper. In her article ("I was sacked for writing about trans censorship") in the UnHerd online publication. Julie recounted the events leading to her sacking, linked closely to the feature piece she wrote on youth gender transition. Julie's article about Australian woman Jay Longanus, who regretted her transition and had sued her psychiatrist was not met kindly in the newsroom where she worked. She described the mood in the newsroom the next day as 'edgy'.

Subsequent developments however have made it difficult for the media to continue its ban on reporting on this issue.

In 2021, an important study[9] published by clinicians, psychiatrists, endocrinologists and psychologists working at Sydney's Westmead Children's Hospital gender service explored the "clinical presentations and challenges" these practitioners had encountered since the clinic opened its doors in 2013.

> They found a patient group with high rates of 'co-morbid' mental conditions, and adverse childhood experiences, including family breakdown and abuse.
>
> The seven authors also describe the clinic as riven and under pressure from 'increasingly dominant, polarised discourses around children with gender dysphoria, including 'emotionally charged, one-sided' media coverage. Some clinicians in the team were more sympathetic to the

---

[8] Julie Szego, "I was sacked for writing about trans censorship. The Australian media has been occupied by activists", *UnHerd*, 19 June 2023.

[9] Kozlowska, K.; McClure, G.; Chudleigh, C.; Maguire, A.M.; Gessler, D.; Scher, S.; Ambler, G.R. "Australian children and adolescents with gender dysphoria: Clinical presentations and challenges experienced by a multidisciplinary team and gender service." Hum. Syst. Ther. Cult. Attach. 2021, 1, 70–95

gender affirmative model, the authors observed, while others sought a more neutral position about their young patients' complex needs.

The media was mixed in the way it reported this study.

The ABC said:[10]

> Some staff have left following the publication of controversial research endorsed by the hospital hierarchy. The research was initiated in 2013 and current frontline staff from the gender unit were not involved.
>
> The research is being weaponised by anti-trans activists and proponents of alternative forms of gender care.
>
> This clash of science, research, and ideology is part of a polarising and sometimes toxic debate over the gender "affirmation" model that's playing out around the world.

In February 2023, these same researchers followed up with a study[11] of 79 young people four to nine years after they first presented at the Westmead clinic. Most of the patients diagnosed with gender dysphoria had ongoing mental health concerns after transitioning. Almost one in 10 dysphoric patients, some who had taken puberty blockers and cross-sex hormones, later discontinued transitioning.

The authors found that the results cast doubt on the central justification for affirmative care, namely that it relieves psychological distress.

However, as Julie Szego recounted, "the response to the Westmead researchers from Australia's pro-affirmation gender medicine fraternity [was] scathing".[12]

Four months after the publication of the Westmead report in 2021, the Royal Australian and New Zealand College of Psychiatrists issued a highly anticipated stance on the treatment of gender dysphoria. This statement[13] underscored the necessity for psychiatrists to conduct thorough mental

---

10 Four Corners, by Patricia Kervelas, Lesley Robinson and Carla Hilderbrand, "Controversial research pulls Westmead children's hospital into centre of fight over gender care", ABC news, posted on 10 July 2023, accessed here: https://www.abc.net.au/news/2023-07-10/transgender-children-westmead-hospital-research-four-corners/102568570

11 Elkadi, J.; Chudleigh, C.; Maguire, A.M.; Ambler, G.R.; Scher, S.; Kozlowska, K. "Developmental Pathway Choices of Young People Presenting to a Gender Service with Gender Distress: A Prospective Follow-Up Study." Children 2023, 10, 314. https://doi.org/10.3390/ children10020314

12 Ibid.

13 The Royal Australian and New Zealand College of Psychiatrists, The role of psychiatrists in working with Trans and Gender Diverse People, Position Statement, December 2023.

health evaluations and to deeply examine an individual's gender identity within the framework of their personal experiences. This development was covered by The Australian.[14]

Regarding the debate on the suitability of a gender-affirmative strategy for minors and adolescents, the College's statement pointed to the significant lack of long-term studies on the results of such approaches. It also recognised the variety of opinions and viewpoints on this matter. Two years earlier, the College had formally supported the RCH's guidelines for affirmative treatment of young individuals, including the use of puberty blockers for those who qualify. The subtle change in the language is notable.

Criticism of the issue or any reporting of these issues was generally labelled or dismissed[15] by gender activists and organisations as 'transphobic', 'extreme', 'far-right bigotry', 'culture wars' etc.

In 2023, the Australian newspaper reported on a call from practitioners for a ban on children receiving gender treatment. The article entitled "Limit kids' access to risky gender drugs"[16] reported on the call from leading psychiatrists to restrict access to puberty blockers for children enrolled in rigorous clinical trials, following studies from Britain that showed that young people's mental health deteriorated while taking the drugs.

In Australia, in August 2022 the Age newspaper reported[17] on the first young person to sue her psychiatrist for professional negligence over the endorsement of hormone therapy and surgeries, Jay Langadinos.

Ms Langadinos sued her psychiatrist for professional negligence over the endorsement of hormone therapy and surgeries. Langadinos' case, reported in August 2022, exemplified the personal and legal complexities of transition regrets, contributing to the broader debate on the adequacy of the gender-affirming approach.

---

14 Natasha Robinson, "Psychiatry body's radical challenge to transgender care", the Australian newspaper, 13 December 2023.

15 Ibid.

16 Rosemary Neill, "UK study finds mental health of one third of kids on puberty blockers deteriorates", *The Australian*, 8 October 2023.

17 Julie Szego, "'Absolutely devastating': woman sues psychiatrist over gender transition", *The Age*, 24 August 2022.

In 2023, the media's engagement with detransitioning stories expanded, notably with Channel 7's Spotlight documentary "The Gender Agenda"[18] in September 2023. The program shared the stories of young people who had undergone gender reassignment surgery and puberty blockers and who subsequently regretted transitioning their gender to share their regrets openly. This was a significant development for mainstream Australian television. Young detransitioners told their stories, and in so doing, pierced the veil that is currently cloaking this entire debate.

The Sydney Morning Herald's "Talking trans"[19] feature in November 2023 further broadened the discourse, presenting an exploration of the experiences of individuals navigating gender dysphoria. This long form opinion article by Michael Bachelard was critical in opening the debate to dissenting voices. By juxtaposing the stories of those who have transitioned positively with those who regret their transitions.

In March 2024, the National Health Service in England announced a ban on puberty blockers for children under the age of 18 years old. This is significant. It received media coverage from all major newspapers and media outlets in Australia. It was reported in the ABC, the Guardian, the Sydney Morning Herald, and the Australian newspaper.

As mainstream media increasingly shows itself willing to report on these issues, including reporting on the testimonies from de-transitioners and concerns raised by practitioners in the field, the hope is that a more informed debate will eventuate.

A transparent and open debate about these important issues is critical if we are to safeguard children and young people (as well as their parents) from making decisions that in many cases are irreversible and make them dependent on lifelong drugs and treatment.

---

18 7 News Spotlight, "Breaking the Silence: The Reality of De-Transitioning", accessed here: https://www.youtube.com/watch?v=JgW_xtIcpew

19 Michael Bachelard, "Talking trans: Adolescents, gender transition and the conversations we need to have", Good Weekend Magazine, Sydney Morning Herald, 25 November 2023.

CHAPTER 11

Dianna Kenny — a practitioner's perspective
- Stories from my practice, clinical studies, and the underlying issues that lead to gender confusion

I was a Professor of Psychology at The University of Sydney, and am now a consulting psychologist, psychotherapist, family therapist, and family dispute resolution practitioner. I have had extensive experience with young people and their families experiencing confusion about their gender.

I am only one of a handful of health professionals in Australia who address underlying issues rather than opt for an automatic "gender affirmation therapy" for young people presenting with gender dysphoria or beliefs that they are transgender. Affirmation therapy includes, but is not limited to, social transitioning such as changing names and pronouns, wearing opposite sex clothing, and medical transitioning such as puberty blockade, cross-sex hormones and surgical procedures.

The American Psychological Association defines "gender identity" as "a person's internal sense of being male, female, or something else". This "something else" has never been adequately defined. All the so-called categories of gender rely on the descriptors "male" and "female."

The concept of "non-binary" which has been accepted so uncritically, is defined as a gender identity that may be both male and female on a sliding scale, neither male nor female, or something else entirely, which again has never been defined.

So far in this book you have read some first-hand accounts of families trying to navigate the fraught waters of gender identity in Australia. In this chapter, I will provide a sample of cases I have dealt with in my practice and offer some of my reflections regarding the factors that have led to gender dysphoria.

I offer them to show that this is happening in a wide range of families and there are always complex underlying reasons. It is poor clinical practice to accept unquestioned a child's declaration that s/he is transgender, yet this is happening in gender clinics, not only in Australia, but internationally. Many young people are set on the path of gender transition after only one or two sessions with a psychiatrist, psychologist, or health professional tasked with determining whether the young person is able to provide informed consent for the potentially life changing procedures that are involved in gender transition.

I hope the following brief cases will provide some insight into the complexity of the psychological difficulties experienced not only by the young person but also their families and the difficult life circumstances that have contributed to the belief that the young person is transgender.

Case 1

A pre-adolescent twelve-year-old boy with an older brother, aged sixteen, suddenly starts wearing makeup and nail polish and demands that his mother buy him female clothing. He declares himself trans. His father is closely attached to his older brother who shares the same interests (racing cars, football, fishing etc) and spends most of his free time with his elder son. He describes his younger son as a "mummy's boy who will probably turn out to be a poofter if he isn't already." This boy tries to resolve his anguish at his father's disdain by defiantly amplifying the dimension of his development so reviled by his father.

Case 2

A young boy who has a younger sister with special needs notices that she receives a lot more parental attention than him. Watching his mother tend to his sister one day, he says "Mummy, will you only love me if I am a girl?" This child makes an error in attending to the wrong dimension as the source of the attention provided to his sister – her gender rather than her disability.

Case 3
A post-pubertal fifteen-year-old female from a Mediterranean family suddenly declares herself transgender. During the assessment, she tells me about her belief that fathers stopped talking to daughters after they started their periods. Her father tells me during a parental assessment that he did not have much in common with his quirky, bookish daughter and found his relationship with his son much easier. This girl wants more of her father's attention and believes she needs to change sex in order to get it.

Case 4
A nineteen-year-old female suddenly announces to her very traditional Indian family that she is transgender. During her psychotherapy, she reveals that her mother makes her feel uncomfortable about her body by constantly referring to her developing female form and stating that it will make a man very happy one day. She has grown up in a highly controlling, overprotective family and panics at the thought of having to marry and have sex with a man.

Case 5
A family of two boys aged six and twelve years old lose their mother after a long illness. Father is a war veteran with PTSD and alcoholism and unable to manage his children's grief. The older boy begins to mercilessly bully his younger brother, who starts to cross-dress, hiding in his mother's wardrobe, and wrapping himself in her clothes. At age twelve, he comes out as transgender, which represents his attempt to merge with his mother, to bring his loved, lost mother back to tend to the gaping emotional wound inside.

Case 6
A fourteen-year-old natal boy first comes out by way of a letter to his parents as 'gay'. He soon changes that declaration to 'bisexual' when he experiences a powerful crush on a female classmate. After she rejects him, he comes out as 'trans' and demands puberty blockers and cross sex hormones. In therapy, his demands for

transition are strident and incessant. He constantly asks me when I am going to tell his parents that he can give consent and go ahead with his transition. He shaves his legs, arms, and body hair, grows his hair long, and starts to wear eye makeup and nail polish. He orders female clothing from the internet and wears it secretly in his room. When his parents confiscate these clothing items, his female friends lend him their own clothes to wear.

Teachers at his school start calling him by his preferred name and pronouns without parental knowledge or permission. Several months after therapy commences, while still vehemently protesting his trans-female identity, he writes a letter to his parents apologising for misleading them. He says he now realises that he was not a trans-female but a 'demigirl' (denoting partial non-binary, partial female gender identity).

He changes this orientation shortly thereafter to 'demiboy', before again writing to his parents, telling them that he was only joking about the whole thing and that they are the only people who have taken it seriously. (This was very far from objective reality). I advised his parents to give their son the opportunity to exit the gender maze without losing face. The next day he asked his parents to take him for a haircut and declared himself 'straight'.

These young people have all had experiences that led them to declare themselves transgender or non-binary. But these declarations represent the symptoms of a complex problem, not the full diagnosis. All these young people, the families who have shared their stories in this book and other Australians deserve to be given appropriate attention and have their underlying issues addressed and dealt with. To place these young people on "affirmative" pathways such as puberty blockade or cross-sex hormones does not address the underlying issues and in fact lead to more complex problems including irreversible physical and psychological harm.

SOCIAL CONTAGION OF GENDER DYSPHORIA

Social contagion is at least partially responsible for the upsurge in gender dysphoria in the past three decades, but this is vehemently denied by most social institutions charged with safeguarding children and young people, including governments, universities and schools, human rights commissions, legal institutions, and sporting bodies.

The misguided adherence to a scientifically bankrupt gender ideology has had, as yet, unfathomed negative impacts on young people, their families, and the wider society. All dispassionate debate is stifled because it would detonate and topple the edifice of gender ideology.

The prevailing view regarding this unprecedented upsurge is that the social and cultural milieu into which the current generation of children and adolescents has been born has permitted disinhibition of expression of their transgendered identity in the same way that left-handedness and homosexuality were permitted freer expression in previous decades, hence leading to increased numbers of those "coming out."

This explanation is unsatisfactory because the asymptotes of the upward surge in left-handed and gay people reach a plateau, unlike the case of gender dysphoria which has shown rapid growth from a very low baseline over the past 30 years. An alternate explanation for this 21st century phenomenon must be canvassed. Social contagion is the prime candidate and evidence strongly suggests that other pathological behaviours, such as eating disorders and self-harm among adolescents also spreads via social contagion, suggesting that gender dysphoria may also be spreading in a similar way.

Social contagion refers to the way that behaviours, beliefs, and attitudes can spread within a community. Studies using extensive data, like the Framingham Heart Study, revealed that social connections strongly influence a wide range of behaviors—such as eating habits, sleep patterns, and substance use – across generations and social networks.

Social network analysis, initially used in public health to trace disease outbreaks, has expanded to investigate the spread of social phenomena through technological advancements and social media. The success of the transgender rights movement in influencing healthcare, education, and legislation is a notable example of an effective network.

MECHANISMS OF SOCIAL CONTAGION

Peer influence

Peers significantly influence each other from an early age, affecting both positive and negative behaviors. During childhood, peer interactions often extend beyond family influence. Gender plays a crucial role in forming peer groups, emphasizing gender norms and identity.

Deviancy Training and co-rumination

Deviancy training, in which deviant behavior is encouraged and rewarded by peers, can lead to antisocial behaviors. Similarly, co-rumination—excessive discussion about problems within peer groups—can exacerbate issues like depression and anxiety. Such dynamics can undermine positive social institutions like schools or treatment programs, highlighting the importance of peer influence in maintaining disordered behaviors.

The challenge of causality

Determining whether peer influence directly causes new behaviors is challenging due to the complexity of social interactions. Adolescents often select peers with similar behaviors, complicating the analysis of peer influence versus peer selection.

Social media's role

Social media platforms, such as Instagram, play a significant role in the spread of mental health issues and potentially harmful behaviors through the mechanism of social contagion. The interactive nature of social media amplifies the spread of information, with both positive and negative effects on mental health.

Evidence of social contagion in gender dysphoria

The concept of social contagion is increasingly supported by evidence of its role in various adolescent psychopathologies, including eating disorders, substance use, and self-harm. The transactivist movement, through its centralized and cohesive networks, has been particularly effective in spreading its message, often resisting dissenting views.

Low gender typicality and peer victimization can significantly impact mental health and social acceptance, leading to higher risks of depression, anxiety, and suicidality. The transgender rights movement has capitalized on these vulnerabilities, offering a sense of belonging and validation for gender non-conforming individuals.

Rapid onset gender dysphoria and social media

The phenomenon of rapid onset gender dysphoria, particularly among adolescent girls, highlights the susceptibility of this demographic to peer and social media influence. The narratives of transgender identity often precede changes in social media consumption, pointing to the role of online communities in shaping identity.

Conclusion

Gender dysphoria and its related ideologies represent a complex social phenomenon that is rapidly spreading, particularly among young people. While our understanding is still evolving, the role of social contagion must be considered in its dissemination across medical, social, and legal spheres. Further research is necessary to fully grasp the implications of this trend.

THE PROBLEM OF ACCURATE DIAGNOSIS AND DESISTANCE

- There are no objective (laboratory, imaging etc) or psychological tests that can reliably diagnose a "true transgender child."
- By adulthood, between 61-98 per cent of children desist from a transgender identity if not medicalized by "gender affirming" treatments. There is no way of predicting who will remain gender dysphoric. Therefore, many children will be irreversibly harmed by gender affirmation therapy.
- PB derail the path of natural desistance – once children are placed on PB, most, as adolescents, progress to cross-sex hormones because of the physiological and/or psychological effects of PBA.
- Watchful waiting with support (and therapy, if indicated) for gender-dysphoric children and adolescents up to the age of 18 years is the gold standard of care worldwide, not gender affirmative therapy.

Comorbid psychiatric conditions

- Psychological conditions co-occurring in up to 75 per cent of young people with gender dysphoria affect their judgement about proceeding with PBA, particularly when these conditions are not properly considered or treated.

CONSEQUENCES OF "GENDER AFFIRMING THERAPY" IN PREPUBERTAL CHILDREN

Infertility

- Puberty blockade (PB) lowers testosterone and estrogen to below normal levels, thus stopping normal puberty. There are no high-quality studies on the short and long-term effects of puberty blockade. Continued suppression of puberty maintains male and female gonads (i.e., sex organs) in a state of immaturity. The later addition of cross sex hormones does not reverse this situation. Involuntary infertility in adults creates psychological distress and depression and reduces quality of life. Infertility is the outcome of puberty suppression. Children do not have the maturity to understand the implications of lifelong infertility.

- Fertility preservation rates are low – fewer than 5 per cent of adolescents attempt cryopreservation.
- Children receiving puberty blockade cannot preserve eggs or sperm. The only options are experimental procedures such as ovarian and testicular tissue cryopreservation.

Impaired sexual function
- Early blockade of puberty stops genital development which results in limited to absent sexual function in adulthood.
- In men, erection, orgasm, and ejaculation are impaired or absent.
- In women, puberty blockade induces menopause and reduces sexual desire.
- Reduced sexual desire in both men and women is associated with decreases in general health and mental wellbeing.

Disruption of normal bone development
- Puberty blockade causes a decline in bone mineral density that may result in early onset osteopenia or osteoporosis.

INFORMED CONSENT

- Children cannot give informed consent to GAT as they cannot fully appreciate the consequences of infertility and loss of sexual function and pleasure, nor the myriad complications of the treatment, including surgical complications if they proceed to breast removal or genital reconstruction.
- Exclusion of parental involvement is dangerous and disrupts the relationships and power balance in the family.

You can read more about this issue and other related topics at my website www.diannakenny.com.au

CHAPTER 12

The international and Australian context

In recent years, the United Kingdom and several Nordic countries, including Sweden, Finland, and Norway, have found themselves at the centre of heated debate surrounding the use of puberty blockers for adolescents experiencing gender dysphoria.

One of the most significant developments in this area of minors and gender identity health care has been the Cass Review, which was commissioned by the National Health Service (NHS) in response to concerns about the long term effects and efficacy of puberty blockers and the sharp increase in the numbers of young people seeking gender treatment. The review was conducted by eminent UK paediatrician Dr Hilary Cass over a four-year period, and the final report was released in March 2024.[20] This comprehensive review has played a pivotal role in reshaping the approach to puberty blockers in these nations.

The Report provides significant evidence of what many of us have suspected all along. Affirmation-only treatments are not best practice and can leave children with irreversible damage.

---

20 CASS Review – Independent Review of Gender Identity Services for Children and Young people. (n.d.). https://cass.independent-review.uk/

Treating children as if they were born in the wrong body denies the fact that most gender incongruent children also experience a range of other issues such as Autism, trauma, depression or eating disorders. The "affirmation-only" models ignore these issues and only attempt to address superficial "gender" changes that make children become medical patients for life.

The primary focus of the Cass Review was on the Gender Identity Development Service (GIDS) at the Tavistock and Portman NHS Foundation Trust, which is the only NHS service in England for children and adolescents experiencing difficulties with their gender identity.

The review explored various aspects of gender identity services, including referral pathways, assessment processes, clinical interventions, safeguarding procedures, and the experiences of service users and their families. It involved gathering evidence from a wide range of sources, including clinicians, service users, families, and other stakeholders.

The review was not about the validity of transgender identities, but rather about the appropriate pathways for children.

The Cass Review identified several key findings regarding the provision of gender identity services for children and young people. The massive increase for services was acknowledged along with long wait times to be assessed. There has been a massive increase in the trend of minors identifying as something they are not. All the while unqualified health practitioners have been prescribing puberty blockers for off label uses.

In speaking with The New Statesman, Dr Cass said[21],

> It's very easy to give people drugs and send them away and find that they're still not able to get out of their bedroom… because you've not looked at the big picture."

> In precocious puberty… what the puberty blockers are doing is returning [abnormally high hormone levels] to normal." But when puberty blockers are used to treat gender-related distress, doctors suppress the normal rise in sex hormones that takes place in adolescence. "It's completely opposite." What's more, when used to treat gender-related distress, blockers are primarily given at a time when the brain is "developing quite complex decision-making abilities and your bones are also growing at pace. So, suppressing at that time is completely different from suppressing in younger children.

---

21 Hannah Barnes, "Hilary Cass: Do I regret doing it? Absolutely not", *The New Statesman Interview*, 8 May 2024.

Concerns were also raised about safeguarding procedures and obtaining informed consent, particularly in cases involving younger children and adolescents. Too often parents are ignored or overwhelmed, or social services intervene blocking parental knowledge and consent.

Based on its findings, the Cass Review made a series of recommendations aimed at improving the provision of gender identity services for children and young people. These recommendations included:

Reducing Waiting Times: Implementing measures to reduce waiting times for assessment and treatment, including increasing capacity within gender identity services and improving referral pathways.

Clinical Governance: Strengthening clinical governance and oversight to ensure that interventions are evidence-based, ethically sound, and in the best interests of the young person.

Support for Families: Providing better support and information for families of trans identified and gender-diverse children and young people, including peer support networks and educational resources.

Research and Training: Investing in research and training to improve understanding of gender identity issues and ensure that healthcare professionals have the necessary knowledge and skills to provide high-quality care.

The recommendations of the Cass Review have already had a significant impact on the provision of gender identity services for children and young people, with the UK, as well as many Nordic countries and some states in the US, ceasing to prescribe puberty blockers and cross sex hormones to minors.

The Gender Identity Development Service (GIDS) at the Tavistock and Portman NHS Foundation Trust have been wound up and minors can no longer be prescribed harmful drugs unless it is under very strict conditions such as a clinical trial.

Watchful waiting pathways have taken on a greater prominence and a whole-health care model implemented. Instead of immediately affirming a child's perceived gender, exploration of underlying issues such as Autism, trauma, depression, eating disorders and other factors will be taken into consideration and addressed.

The NHS and relevant medical bodies have begun to revisit guidelines and protocols, emphasising a more cautious approach and stressing the importance of comprehensive assessments before initiating such treatments.[22]

Simultaneously, Sweden,[23] Finland,[24] and Norway[25] closely monitored the developments in the UK and embarked on their own reviews of existing practices. Concerns regarding the potential impact of puberty blockers on physical and psychological well-being led these nations to reconsider the widespread use of these interventions. The emphasis shifted towards a more individualised approach, prioritising thorough assessments, mental health support, and a careful consideration of the risks and benefits before recommending puberty blockers.

At the time of writing Australian politicians have ignored or rejected the review. Some have made statements that the recommendations will be taken into consideration in due time but no actions have yet been taken.

In general however, Australia is pushing ahead with draconian and harmful legislation that enshrines the "affirmation-only" model of dealing with gender incongruent minors.

One of the fundamental shifts in Australian law has been the recognition of gender identity. Several states and territories have enacted legislation allowing individuals to change the gender marker on their official documents to reflect their 'affirmed' gender identity without requiring surgery.

It is now legal in most states of Australia to rewrite historical facts regarding a person's sex at birth. Instead of reflecting biological reality, birth certificates can now be changed to mirror a person's feelings, and they can be changed every 12 months if desired. Victoria[26] led the charge

---

22 Producer, B. L. M. L. C. &. J. P. L. (2023, June 9). Puberty blockers to be given only in clinical research. BBC News. https://www.bbc.com/news/uk-65860272

23 Sweden's Karolinska ends all use of puberty blockers and Cross-Sex hormones for minors outside of clinical studies. (n.d.). SEGM. https://segm.org/Sweden_ends_use_of_Dutch_protocol

24 One Year Since Finland Broke with WPATH "Standards of Care." (n.d.). SEGM. https://segm.org/Finland_deviates_from_WPATH_prioritizing_psychotherapy_no_surgery_for_minors

25 Cohen, J. (2023, June 6). Increasing number of European nations adopt a more cautious approach to Gender-Affirming care among minors. Forbes. https://www.forbes.com/sites/joshuacohen/2023/06/06/increasing-number-of-european-nations-adopt-a-more-cautious-approach-to-gender-affirming-care-among-minors/?sh=11a0b0367efb

26 Change or Suppression (Conversion) Practices Prohibition Act 2021. (n.d.). https://www.legislation.vic.gov.au/as-made/acts/change-or-suppression-conversion-practices-prohibition-act-2021

followed by Queensland[27] and Tasmania.[28] Western Australia[29] and NSW[30] are considering self-identification laws as we write.

Many states have also criminalised opposition to gender identity ideology. In Victoria for example it is unlawful to pray for gender incongruent people to accept their natal sex or for a medical practitioner to recommend anything other than 'affirmation' therapy. In Queensland for example, women's only gyms must now accept males who claim to be female.[31]

In 2013, as one of her last acts as Prime Minister, Julia Gillard removed sex-based protections from the *Sex Discrimination Act 1984* (SDA).[32] It sounds like something straight out of George Orwell's dystopian novel '1984'. The Gillard government removed definitions of male and female, replacing the terms with 'anyone who identifies' as male or female.

This has put sex and gender identity on an equal footing under the law but in direct opposition to each other. Sex relies on biological reality, whereas gender identity denies it.

Tickle v Giggle[33] is a landmark Federal Court judgment handed down in Australia in 2024. Sall Grover, CEO and owner of female-only app Giggle, refused access to Roxy Tickle, a male who identifies as a woman. Ms Grover claimed she could exclude him based on his sex, but he argued that she couldn't, based on his gender identity. The Federal Court decided in his favour, finding no direct discrimination, but rather that Tickle experienced 'indirect discrimination'. Justice Bromwich found that "sex is changeable"

---

27 Queensland, S. O. (2023, June 14). New laws passed to modernise birth certificates. Ministerial Media Statements. https://statements.qld.gov.au/statements/97953

28 Births, Deaths and Marriages: Gender registration. (n.d.). https://www.justice.tas.gov.au/bdm/gender-registration#:
~:text=The%20parents%20or%20guardians%20of%20a%20child%20can,
registration%20of%20gender%20is%20approved%20by%20a%20magistrate.

29 Reforming sex and gender recognition laws in Western Australia | Western Australian Government. (n.d.). Western Australian Government. https://www.wa.gov.au/government/media-statements/McGowan-Labor-Government/Reforming-sex-and-gender-recognition-laws-in-Western-Australia-20221221

30 A new equality bill. (n.d.). Alex Greenwich. https://www.alexgreenwich.com/equality_bill

31 Gender identity and your rights. (n.d.). https://www.qhrc.qld.gov.au/your-rights/for-lgbtiq-people/gender-identity-and-your-rights

32 Sex Discrimination Act 1984. https://www.legislation.gov.au/C2004A02868/latest/text

33 Tickle v Giggle for Girls Pty Ltd (No.2) [2024] FCA 960.

and non-binary and held that "the concept of sex has broadened over the 30 years since the SDA". Ms Grover was ordered to pay $10,000 in compensation as well as legal costs. On 3 October 2024, Ms Grover announced[34] that she was appealing the decision. The outcome of this appeal will be critical for the protection of sex-based rights in Australia.

Access to gender-affirming healthcare has been a focal point in the legal discourse surrounding transgender rights. Calling drugs and surgery 'affirming' care is to employ Orwellian language, as it means the exact opposite. Puberty blockers, cross-sex hormones and surgery all serve to deny a person's gender and enable them to appropriate the stereotypes of the opposite sex.

So-called gender 'affirming' care means prescribing puberty blockers to minors, despite the drugs being used off-label. They have never been tested, studied or approved for such use. While the UK and Nordic nations recognise the potential harm of these drugs and have wound back their programs, Australia is pushing aggressively ahead, even criminalising opposition to the model.

Many politicians have falsely described 'wait-and-watch' approaches as "conversion therapy", while states like Victoria have taken specific steps to protect transgender individuals from what they claim are harmful conversion practices. Legislation has been introduced to prohibit any attempt to change or suppress a person's gender identity, denying medical practitioners the ability to comprehensively address underlying issues such as Autism, trauma or depression. Parents are threatened with having their children removed from their custody if they refuse to 'affirm' their child and Christians are told they cannot pray for individuals to embrace their biological reality if they want to 'convert' to the opposite sex.

Medical practitioners are too afraid to oppose the legislation, so they either refer patients on or reluctantly go along with the 'affirmation' model. Dr Jillian Spencer, a senior psychiatrist at the Queensland Children's Hospital, was stood down after being branded 'transphobic.'[35] All she did

---

34 Joanna Panagopoulos, "Sall Grover appeals landmark transgender discrimination win", The Australian, 3 October 2024, accessed here: https://www.theaustralian.com.au/nation/sall-grover-appeals-landmark-transgender-discrimination-win/news-story/8268abfb20ea13ad02d01ef643a978b

35 Adf. (2023, July 27). Australian Doctors Federation statement on the independence of medical decision making. Australian Doctors Federation. https://ausdoctorsfederation.org.au/2023/07/26/australian-doctors-federation-statement-on-the-independence-of-medical-decision-making/

was merely rely on her medical expertise to point out the lack of data and evidence for the affirmation model and share her concerns about the serious side-effects of puberty blockers. These drugs can cause catastrophic, irreversible side effects such as sterility, no sexual function, brain and bone development issues. It is more than reasonable to question the prescribing of these drugs to children who cannot possibly consent to the dire consequences of taking them.

Jasmine Sussex, a breastfeeding expert with more than 20 years, was sacked from her volunteer position with the Australian Breastfeeding Association for refusing to call women chest-feeders instead of breast-feeders and not moving on the fact that men cannot and should not breastfeed.[36]

Efforts to create inclusive environments for transgender individuals extend into education policies. Some states have implemented guidelines and frameworks to promote inclusivity and respect for diverse gender identities within educational institutions. A myriad of celebration days exist and staff or students who object are vilified. Gender identity ideology has infiltrated every subject and school culture to the point that gender diverse children are granted special protections and privileges. In states like Victoria, staff can socially transition children without parental knowledge or consent.

Former teacher Moira Deeming, a democratically elected MP, was thrown out of her parliamentary party for her efforts to champion female-sex based rights. After attending a public rally called Let Women Speak, which she informed the government and her party beforehand that she would do, she was falsely smeared a Nazi and removed from the party room. Having to serve on the back bench she has fought hard for an apology and reinstatement. John Pesutto, the Liberal Party leader of Victoria, and his leadership team have continued to brand Moira a Nazi and she has now begun defamation proceedings against them.[37]

---

36 Australian Breastfeeding Association investigate counsellors for using term 'mother' (2022, May 9). [Video]. Skynews. https://www.skynews.com.au/opinion/rita-panahi/australian-breastfeeding-association-investigate-counsellors-for-using-term-mother/video/b1e08943cf14167e19bd92dbf4f3694a

37 Godde, C. (2024, February 2). "Moira Deeming and John Pesutto defamation trial procedural hearing". Nine News.https://www.9news.com.au/national/victoria-moira-deeming-john-pesutto-defamation-trial-procedural-hearing/16763c04-5623-48d5-bf4b-bb256354f175

Hobart City Councillor Louise Elliot has been harassed, suspended and referred to the anti-discrimination board for a speech she made at the Let Women Speak event in Tasmania. She said "transwomen are transwomen and remain men." That is an unarguable fact. No one can change their sex. Men cannot become women. Only men can be transwomen. Yet Louise now has to defend her words before a tribunal because the truth has upset a few activists.[38]

The world of academia is also under siege. Associate Professor Holly-Lawford Smith has been constantly harassed on campus at Melbourne University where she teaches feminism.[39] Students who are upset with her stance that men cannot be women intimidate her students, graffiti the grounds and make threats toward her. All for upholding scientific, biological reality.

The Australian Sports Commission released guidelines for transgender inclusion that have been adopted by almost every sporting code in Australia.[40] The SDA makes it clear that discrimination can legally occur if it is proven that biological advantage exists or if there is potential harm to females by including males in their divisions. The frustrating thing is most sporting codes are preferring 'inclusion' of males in female divisions rather than safety and fairness for female athletes.

Many codes have taken it a step further, introducing sanctions or fines, suspension or expulsion for players, parents, coaches or officials who object to such policies. Most community clubs can not afford the drama and legal costs of such battles, so they suck it up and refuse to take on the goliaths that run the show.

I have been on the sharp end of that stick with three applications for apprehension of violence orders (AVO) against me for identifying two males in female soccer competitions.

A staff member from Football Australia applied but withdrew before it went to court. Another player had NSW Police apply for an AVO, but

---

38 Evans, L. (2023, November 15). 'Bring it on': Councillor faces legal battle over transgender comments. Skynews. https://www.skynews.com.au/australia-news/hobart-city-councillor-louise-elliot-to-face-tribunal-inquiry-over-comments-she-made-about-transgender-women-earlier-this-year/news-story/067c44293d752c2d611cc182381376e0

39 Grand, C. L. (2023, May 20). University closes book on lecturer transphobia complaints. The Sydney Morning Herald. https://www.smh.com.au/national/university-closes-book-on-lecturer-transphobia-complaints-20230518-p5d9c4.html

40 Trans and gender diverse inclusion. (n.d.). Australian Sports Commission. https://www.sportaus.gov.au/integrity_in_sport/transgender_and_gender_diverse_people_in_sport

after six months of mentions in court, and tens of thousands of dollars, they withdrew the moment it went to hearing before a magistrate in Burwood local court.

A third private AVO was applied for by another player. That went to hearing and the application was denied. The process was the punishment, tying us up in expensive legal proceedings for ten months.

Both players also filed vilification complaints against me for referring to them as male. The NSW anti-discrimination board referred the cases to the NSW Civil and Administrative Tribunal but the NSW Attorney-General intervened and the cases were dismissed.[41] As the spokeswoman for Binary, a registered third-party political campaigner, I have the right to implied freedom of political speech. If anyone wants to argue that it must be done in court that comes under federal jurisdiction as it is under constitutional law.

The point is, the process is the punishment. All of these legal actions are designed to syphon funds from campaigns and wear us down. They hope we will be sufficiently intimidated and silenced.

This is just a snapshot of the state of affairs in Australia.

This book is about giving families who are victims of gender identity ideology a voice and a platform to tell their stories. They are victims of the legislation, the medical industry and the education system that has let them down.

---

41 Blanch v Smith, NSW Caselaw. (n.d.). https://www.caselaw.nsw.gov.au/decision/18d1fa80234887e14599829f

CHAPTER 13
Resources for families

Navigating the complexities and misinformation surrounding the trans issue can be incredibly distressing for friends and family of trans youth. There's no question that loving parents want the best for their children, yet in a world where even the most trusted institutions have been captured by gender ideology, exactly what it means to be 'loving' has become blurred.

Does love always mean affirmation? (Hint: NO!). Couldn't there be other underlying issues contributing to their obsession over gender? (Hint: YES!). Aren't children and adolescents too young to make life-altering medical decisions like the loss of fertility? Shouldn't I be allowed to ask them to wait? (Hint: YES!).

Many parents would be shocked to discover that questions like these are now illegal in states like Victoria under the charge of 'conversion and suppression' practices.

Despite the pressure and misinformation, it's vital parents understand that having compassion doesn't have to mean 100 per cent agreeing with their beliefs, or condoning their behaviour.

Many de-transitioners (former trans-identifying people) caution parents of gender dysphoric children against simply presenting scientific facts and arguments about biological sex. While truth is certainly on your side, there are complex layers underlying the gender issue meaning a guns-blazing approach is likely to drive them further down the ideological hole.

It's important to prioritise building a quality relationship with your child and moving the conversation away from gender and transitioning as much as it's possible. Remember that studies show around 90 per cent of children will grow out of their gender dysphoria if left to go through normal puberty.

Many young women who were caught up in the transgender craze in their teenage years describe body image issues, unrealistic expectations of womanhood, and a hypersexualised culture as contributing factors that led to their trans identity. Parents play an important role in combating these negative cultural messages and engaging in constructive conversations around some of these damaging lies they may be believing. Flaunting your body and liking 'girly things' do not make a woman, nor do muscles and cars make a man. Gender ideology is purely based on stereotypes and denies the beautiful diversity of character and temperament of males and females.

TIPS FOR FINDING A TRUSTWORTHY THERAPIST

Extract from Parents of Rapid Onset Gender Dysphoria website[42], a support group for parents.

> Gender dysphoria is a complex and multi-faceted issue that can be caused by many factors. Unfortunately, it is difficult to find a therapist who understands this. Many therapists will simply "affirm" your child and set them on the path to social and medical transition.
>
> It is essential to find a therapist who will take a more cautious, psychologically-informed approach to your child. They must take the time to truly understand your child and explore the roots of their dysphoria. And they must be willing to consider healthier, less-invasive alternatives for dealing with your child's dysphoria before resorting to social and/or medical transitioning.
>
> To that end, here are a set of guidelines to help you find a therapist you can trust.
>
> DO NOT take them to any therapist who claims to specialise in 'gender identity,' 'gender dysphoria' or purports to help those who are 'questioning their gender identity'.

---

[42] Read more on the website at www.parentsofrogdkids.com

These therapists are likely to simply affirm your child and encourage them to persist in their belief without ever questioning why they may feel this way. In some cases, such therapists have recommended social and medical transition after as little as one visit. We have even heard reports of therapists recommending this over the phone without ever having met the child.

Choose an experienced therapist (minimum 10 years) who has a large population of adolescent and young adult patients, especially young girls.

They are most likely to be noticing that a lot of their patients are suddenly deciding they are trans and may already be growing suspicious.

Be proactive. Help them to learn about this dangerous trend by bringing them helpful, authoritative articles, such as:

"Gender Dysphoria is Not One Thing" written by Drs. Bailey and Blanchard, two of the world's most respected researchers in gender dysphoria,

"Rapid-Onset Gender Dysphoria in Adolescents and Young Adults", Dr. Lisa Littman's groundbreaking new study, and

"Rapid-onset gender dysphoria in adolescents stirs debate" posted in MedScape.

Ask them to watch and consider some testimonies of detransitioners and desisters who are very insightful and highlight the underlying issues that should be addressed.

Before you allow your child to spend any time alone with a therapist, prescreen them by asking them open-ended questions to learn their approach towards gender dysphoric kids.

Really listen to their answers. This should give you a very good idea of their approach.

If they act insulted that you would dare to question them, leave.

If they refuse to tell you their approach, leave.

If they tell you they will 'affirm' your child, or 'let the child be their guide', leave.

Be extremely wary of any therapist who intentionally excludes the parents from the child's therapy and insists on only seeing the child alone. They may be encouraging your child behind your back. (We have even heard reports of this - and it was at a major children's hospital.)

Find a therapist who is willing to involve the parents - at times - as part of the therapy. Gender dysphoria can have roots in the family dynamic, so it is important to find a therapist who is willing to take this into consideration.

Explore our website www.binary.org.au for more resources and videos. Inform yourself about the serious medical consequences and side effects children experience who take puberty blockers and cross sex hormones.

Engage with your child's school and make sure you know what they are being taught and exposed to while not in your care. Check their library books and ask to speak with head teachers or school principals if you are concerned. Do it frequently and build a solid relationship with school leaders. Join the parent groups and don't assume your child will tell you every little detail of what they are exposed to during school hours.

Monitor their screen use and exposure to social media and especially chat groups. We have heard over and over again about children being curious and then being groomed online via chat groups. Children who are on the spectrum or ostracised at school appear to be extremely vulnerable. These chat groups, and activists within the school community, offer lonely and isolated children an identity that is celebrated, often with special privileges attached.

Check council run libraries for inappropriate content. Borrow the books and take them to public council meetings to show the councillors how damaging and harmful such content is.

Remember that puberty is a difficult rite of passage for everyone, but it is a human right. Be as supportive as possible by forming a strong relationship with your child. Eat meals together or do special activities that they enjoy to foster trust and open communication. Gender confusion is a part of the search for identity and worth. Continually reassure your child they are loved, valued, wanted and enough. Build their confidence as you find resources and pathways to fan into flame their strengths and support them in their weaknesses. Reach out to other parents for support and build a community that is safe for your child to be themselves.

There are many excellent books to read and documentaries to watch that can remind you that you are not alone. There are also some support networks in Australia that we can help connect you into. Many are not public because of some people's need for privacy and to protect them from potential backlash.

RECOMMENDED READING

Abigail Shrier, **Irreversible Damage: The Transgender Craze Seducing Our Daughters**, Regnery Publishing, 2020.

Kathleen Stock, **Material Girls, Why Reality Matters for Feminism**, Fleet, 1st edition, 2022.

Helen Joyce, **Trans, When Ideology Meets Reality**, Oneworld Publications, 2021.

Bernard Lane "Gender Clinic News" Substack[43]

DOCUMENTARIES

What is a Woman? Presented by Matt Walsh on The Daily Wire[44]

Detrans by Prager on youtube.com[45]

The Wounds That Won't Heal, EP 319 - Detransitioner Chloe Cole[46] interviewed by Jordan B Peterson on youtube.com

---

43 https://substack.com/@genderclinicnews
44 https://www.dailywire.com/videos/what-is-a-woman
45 https://www.youtube.com/watch?v=3yvjFSX0TB0
46 https://www.youtube.com/watch?v=6O3MzPeomqs

CHAPTER 14

The future for our children

I don't know about you, but I have found these stories extremely harrowing to read. I can't imagine how difficult it is for these brave families who have shared their stories in the hope of helping others who may face similar circumstances.

These stories only scratch the surface of the tragedy unfolding across our nation.

It is an avoidable tragedy.

These families have suffered needlessly as a result of politicians legislating lies and appeasing a small minority. The impact has been catastrophic and pervasive. Thousands of young people have been lied to. It will take decades to reverse the dreadful consequences.

But with stories like the ones in this book, politicians will have to sit up and take notice. They are ultimately the ones responsible for creating the perfect storm for vulnerable youth in our country.

They, or their predecessors, have legislated lies that have negatively impacted the health system, the education system and social services system.

Julia Gillard's government set it all in motion in 2013 when it removed protections for sex from the Sex Discrimination Act.

As a result we are confronted with the nonsensical and utterly ridiculous notion that "anyone who identifies as a woman is a woman." You can't identify as something that is not defined.

A woman is an adult human female. 'Female' is a scientific term that denotes a body with female xx chromosomes and a body with a reproductive system geared around producing large gametes (eggs).

Sex is an immutable fact, not something assigned at birth, not something that can be changed. Costumes, drugs and surgery do not negate the sex of a person's body. Sex is written on every single cell that contains a nucleus in our bodies.

The Sex Discrimination Act should provide protections for sex-based rights. But it doesn't. It has been rendered impotent by the inclusion of gender identity. Gender identity is based on feelings, a personal expression if you like. It is changeable, immeasurable, without bounds, without standards. It is not something that should qualify in law.

We have spent decades trying to dismantle sex stereotypes and now we have undone all that hard work by enforcing the stereotypes via appropriation! It is insane and dangerous.

Every federal and state government since 2013 has incrementally changed laws to protect and promote those few individuals who refuse to accept their true identities. Politicians have pandered to the lie that a person can change their sex. They want to appear 'kind' and 'tolerant' but have in fact created a situation that is cruel and full of harm.

States have changed identity laws to allow people to rewrite historical facts on their birth certificates and other official identity documents. They have allowed males to gain access to female spaces without regard for the way these policies impacts female sex-based rights.

Males who are addicted to pornography are being granted the ability to live out their fantasies in public and force everyone else to comply.

Vulnerable young girls who are already struggling with body image are being offered false solutions to avoid the horror of being sexualised or marginalised because they don't fit the stereotypes. Meanwhile males who are obsessed with female stereotypes are being given free reign to dress and act in hypersexualised ways and insist the world view them as female.

Autistic, traumatised, depressed and vulnerable children are not being offered comprehensive treatments to enable them to cope, endure or overcome. Instead, they are immediately put onto discredited "affirmation" pathways that lock them into being life-long medical industry consumers – who still suffer with their underlying issues. Now many are dealing with the completely avoidable regret of having subjected their bodies to experimental drugs and surgeries. It is devastating!

The only way we will achieve real change is to lobby those in power who write the laws. The politicians need to hear these stories and be held to account. They have the ability to rewrite bad laws and save a generation from more harm.

Politicians need to read the stories of and meet people and families like the ones in this book. Daughters who have been snatched from their loving families to face a depressed and uncertain future without their breasts, suffering male pattern baldness and atrophied wombs.

They need to be confronted with the families torn apart by adult males fulfilling their fantasies while leading their children down the same dark pathways.

They need to meet the heartbroken mothers who have been sidelined by a health and education system that has no regard for parental knowledge or consent.

Make sure your local MPs and Senators, both state and federal, hear about or read these stories. Get them a copy of the book, make an appointment to see them. Make sure they are without excuse. The heartbreak of the families in this book is the heartbreak of our nation.

Despite the devastation these families have endured, there is hope.

The Cass Review and the fact that countries such as the UK, some states in the US and many Nordic countries have banned these harmful practices cannot be avoided much longer. These and other important studies need to be shared widely. They are comprehensive and evidence-based. They contain important facts to counter the false narrative that a person can change their sex.

Politicians, media personalities and people in influential positions need to be asked hard questions and we must demand real answers.

"What is a woman" is not a gotcha question, but a valid and fundamental question that must be answered honestly, and backed with evidence. The answer to this question must inform policy and law for all our sakes. The answer to the question is a line that cannot be moved, unlike the inexplicable concept of gender identity.

Safeguarding children must be addressed and prioritised. The hypersexualised culture we live in puts so many young people at risk. Unsupervised access to the internet is a recipe for disaster as families in this book have testified. Children should not be exposed to sexualised content in public or school libraries.

Lying to children, or indeed to anyone, and claiming they can change their sex is an abomination. We must all do the hard work of affirming children and encouraging them to accept who they are. We must teach them to be resilient and to overcome trials and difficult circumstances.

We would never "affirm" a child's eating disorder by giving them liposuction and allowing them to starve themselves. We would never "affirm" an addictive personality with alcohol or gambling. We would never "affirm" a depressed person with drugs or self-harm.

We must confront and stop these "affirmation" practices of gender identity that are based on lies and unachievable promises. Regardless of what measures these children take, they will never become the opposite sex or without sex. They are what they are. The only kind thing to do is to come alongside them and help them accept the truth and reality of who they are. They must endure puberty to mature. They must embrace the facts to thrive.

No child is born in the wrong body. Every child is a unique and beautiful creation, designed to add colour to our world in a way only that individual can. Their unique attributes need to be fanned into flame, for their sake and for ours. We all need each other for a thriving society to exist. When children are abused and misled it is a shame on us all.

The laws of nature dictate that there must be resistance in order for something to become strong. Muscles can only grow when they are forced to cope with resistance. The strongest trees have deep roots after being buffeted by wind and the elements to make them strong.

Our children do not need superficial, false or misleading treatments to help them avoid difficult situations or periods of life. They need us to come alongside them and lead them through the storms they will face. Together we can face the resistance and become strong.

It should never be an option to medicate them into accepting a lie. It should never be an option to separate a child from their loving family to appease some activists and affirm their delusion.

Most importantly our society must be focused on loving and reassuring young people based on truth.

Unspeakable tragedies happen. Trauma is inflicted on the innocent. Our minds play tricks on us. As humans we are very prone to confusion. Trying to escape our problems is a common-to-all experience.

But there is a plumb line, a true north; unarguable evidence that we can all rely on.

Sex is binary.

There is only male or female. No other option. No third gamete.

There are certainly disorders when it comes to biological sex, but these do not negate the fact there is still only male or female. Disorders include but are not limited to males with female sex characteristics, females with male sex characteristics, and non-functioning reproductive systems that still contain elements of either male or female.

Male or female, that's all folks.

When we admit the truth, we can right the wrongs and face reality. It was a gross mistake to legislate the lie that people can change their sex. The consequences have been absolutely devastating for too many. The mop up will take years, even decades as broken people and families pick up the pieces.

Gender identity is like an uncontainable mist. It has no substance. It moves and evaporates when the sun shines. When we shine the light onto gender ideology, we see the truth – sex is binary and immutable.

Our sincere hope in publishing this book is to shine a light on the experiences of ordinary families in Australia who have been impacted so profoundly by radical gender ideology. Gender ideology is no longer just an obscure radical theory thought up by academics – it has made its way into our schools, our families, and into our children's psyches.

For far too long, the voices and questions of parents and families have been dismissed, silenced, hidden, and ridiculed. So many of the parents describe having no one to confide in when navigating this most complex of issues concerning their children.

And the impacts have been devastating.

We can never say thank you enough to the brave people who have shared their personal stories with us in these pages. They are real people, who are devastated, who are hurting and living with great pain or regret, who are now in some cases thriving and living with the acceptance of their situation, and some who are still hoping for a brighter day.

And we are so proud to provide a platform where their stories can at last be shared.

We know that their stories are multiplied thousands of times over in Australia alone.

It is our hope that other parents reading this book will know they are not alone.

Our hope also is this book will be a tool to effect change. We must continue to educate the public and raise awareness with politicians. We must not stop until the Sex Discrimination Act once again contains a definition and protections for sex-based rights.

We must offer support, compassion and hope to those impacted by gender ideology. Nearly everyone has a story of someone they know who has been captured by gender ideology. So many sad stories based on false narratives and promises that cannot possibly be realised.

We can all be a part of the change and influence our culture for good. Anytime someone tries to silence you, remember these stories. Stand firm, speak up and speak loudly for those whose voice has been stolen from them.

Truth, reality and evidence-based science will prevail. It is just a matter of time and a commitment from each one of us to stay the course.

www.ingramcontent.com/pod-product-compliance
Lightning Source LLC
Chambersburg PA
CBHW022015290426
44109CB00015B/1179